Peate's Body Systems

Peate's Body Systems

The Skin

Ian Peate, OBE FRCN EN(G) RGN DipN(Lond) RNT BEd(Hons) MA(Lond) LLM

Editor in Chief, British Journal of Nursing;
Consultant Editor, Journal of Paramedic Practice;
Consultant Editor, International Journal for Advancing Practice;
Visiting Professor, Northumbria University;
Visiting Professor, Buckinghamshire New University;
Professorial Fellow, University of Roehampton;
Visiting Senior Clinical Fellow, University of Hertfordshire

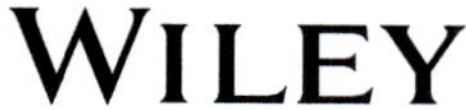

Library of Congress Cataloging-in-Publication Data

Names: Peate, Ian, author.
Title: The skin / Ian Peate, OBE FRCN EN(G), RGN DipN(Lond), RNT Bed BEd (Hons), MA(Lond) LLM; editor in chief, British Journal of Nursing; Consultant Editor, Journal of Paramedic Practice; Consultant Editor, International Journal for Advancing Practice; Visiting Professor, Northumbria University, Visiting Professor, St Georges University of London and Kingston University London, Professorial Fellow, Roehampton University; Visiting Senior Clinical Fellow, University of Hertfordshire.
Description: Hoboken, NJ : John Wiley & Sons, 2025. | Series: Peate's body systems | Includes bibliographical references and index.
Identifiers: LCCN 2024041162 | ISBN 9781394252626 (paperback) | ISBN 9781394252633 (epub) | ISBN 9781394252640 (adobe pdf)
Subjects: LCSH: Dermatology–Textbooks. | Skin–Anatomy–Textbooks.
Classification: LCC RL71 .P38 2025
LC record available at https://lccn.loc.gov/2024041162

Cover Images: © marinashevchenko/Adobe Stock, © phototechno/Getty Images, © 4luck/Adobe Stock, © Oleksandr Pokusai/Adobe Stock
Cover Design: Wiley

Set in 9.5pt STIXTwo by Lumina Datamatics
Printed and bound by CPI Group (UK) Ltd, Croydon, CR0 4YY

C9781394252626_200125

Contents

Preface

Welcome to *Peate's Body Systems*; there are 12 books in the series. This is a comprehensive collection of textbooks designed to support and enrich the knowledge of health and care workers across various fields. This series is intended to be a valuable resource for those who are dedicated to understanding the intricacies of human biology, physiology and the various systems that sustain life.

Peate's Body Systems series is rooted in the belief that a deep and thorough understanding of the human body is essential for providing the highest standard of care. Each book in this series is thoroughly crafted to offer clear, accurate and up-to-date information on different body systems. The aim is to bridge the gap between complex scientific concepts and practical, everyday applications in healthcare settings.

PURPOSE AND SCOPE

The purpose of this series is to provide health and care workers with:

- Foundational knowledge, with explanations of the anatomical structures and physiological functions of the body systems

- Insights into how these systems interact with each other and how they are impacted by various diseases and conditions, highlighting clinical relevance and encouraging practical application

STRUCTURE OF THE SERIES

Each book in *Peate's Body Systems* focuses on a specific body system:

The Cardiovascular System	The Female Reproductive System
The Respiratory System	The Male Reproductive System
The Digestive System	The Musculoskeletal System
The Renal System	The Skin
The Nervous System	The Ear, Nose and Throat
The Endocrine System	The Eyes

Every chapter is designed to be comprehensive yet accessible, making complex information easier to digest and apply. Figures, tables, boxes, illustrations and flowcharts have been extensively used to support visual learning and reinforce key concepts.

This series is tailored for:

- Healthcare students: those in nursing and allied health programmes

- Practicing professionals: nurses, therapists and other care workers seeking to deepen their understanding and stay current with the latest developments in health and care

- Educators and trainers: educators who require reliable and comprehensive teaching materials to advise and instruct the next generation of healthcare providers

Commitment to Excellence. The series is committed to providing quality educational resources that not only inform but also inspire and empower health and care workers. By equipping you with a robust understanding of the systems of life, you will be better prepared to make informed decisions, deliver compassionate care and ultimately improve patient outcomes.

Thank you for choosing *Peate's Body Systems* as your trusted resource. I hope these textbooks serve as a valuable tool in your ongoing journey of learning and professional development.

IAN PEATE
London

Acknowledgements

I would like to acknowledge the help and support of my partner Jussi Lahtinen. Acknowledgements also go to staff at the RCN Library in London. My thanks go to Tom Marriott, Christabel Daniel Raj, Bhavya Boopathi and all those at Wiley.

Anatomy and Physiology of the Skin

CHAPTER 1

The skin or integumentary system functions as an important shield for the body, ensuring its survival using a range of protective mechanisms. Without skin and its protective mechanisms, the human being would not survive. The skin's constant visibility allows it to reflect both our emotional and physiological states, such as blushing or cyanosis (Stephens 2021). Given its constant exposure, the skin is highly prone to diseases and infections, despite its near-complete waterproof nature.

SKIN

HOMEOSTASIS

The skin has a multifaceted role in maintaining homeostasis and safeguarding overall health. Homeostasis refers to the body's ability to maintain stability and balance amidst changing external and internal conditions (Evans 2022). Within the context of the skin, homeostasis manifests in various ways, notably in regulating body temperature. The body is constantly striving to keep its internal environment within a narrow range that is conducive to optimal function. When exposed to heat, such as on a hot day, the skin carefully works to dissipate excess heat through mechanisms such as sweating, thereby preventing overheating and maintaining equilibrium.

The skin appendages are specialised structures derived from the skin itself, each serving a unique purpose. They are integral to the skin's function. Hair follicles, sweat glands and sebaceous glands are among the significant appendages, each contributing to the skin's protective and regulatory functions. Sweat glands, for example, act as a coolant, secreting sweat to cool the body during physical exertion or exposure to high temperatures.

An adult possesses a skin surface area ranging from 1.5 to 2 m^2, weighing roughly 4.1 kg, which surpasses the weight of the brain twofold. Within this vast expanse, an intricate network thrives. There are approximately 4.5 million blood vessels, 3.6 million nerves, 2.6 million sweat glands, 1500 sensory receptors and over 3 million cells undergoing continuous turnover (Peate 2020). Notably, the skin commands a significant portion of the body's circulatory resources, receiving nearly one-third of the total blood flow (McLaughlin 2018).

Moving away from the numbers associated with the skin, the profound influence of the skin on human health and well-being is important. Much like the bricks and mortar of a sturdy house, the skin forms a resilient framework that shields the body from external attacks. The skin fends off environmental hazards and microbial invaders. Its protective competence reaches beyond mere physical barriers, incorporating complex immune mechanisms that safeguard against the harmful effects of pathogens and foreign substances.

The importance of the skin extends beyond safeguarding the body; it serves as a hub of sensory experiences, facilitating tactile sensations and emotional expressions. The delight of a gentle touch and the comfort of an affectionate hug are all facilitated by the skin's intricate

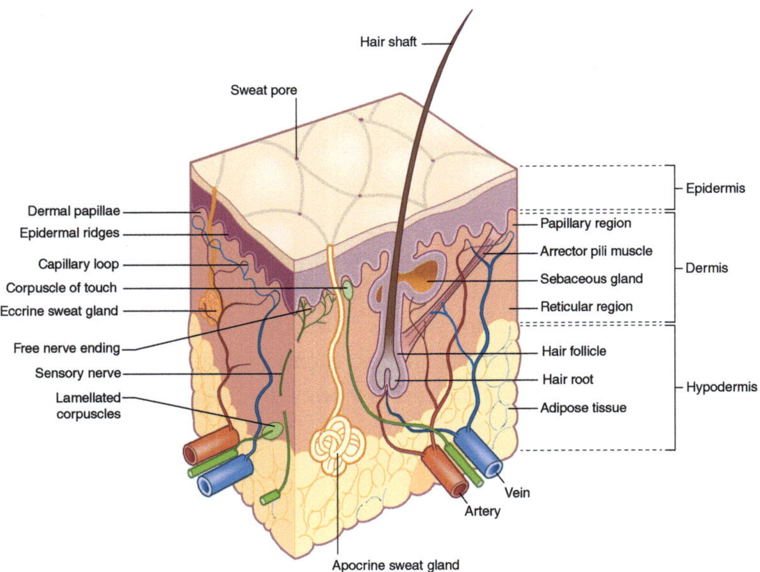

FIGURE 1.1   The skin and associated structures

array of receptors. The skin has the ability to allow a person to experience pleasure, pain and other stimuli from the external environment (Peate 2019).

Any disruption in the skin's integrity can bring on a cascade of physical and psychological repercussions, highlighting its indispensable role in preserving quality of life. Whether it is a minor cut or a long-standing skin condition, the repercussions extend well beyond the skin's surface, impacting our overall well-being.

The skin transcends its superficial appearance; it represents a remarkable feat of biological engineering, intricately integrated into the essence of human existence. Exploring the skin's intricacies further, our appreciation for this steadfast protector grows, as it diligently maintains the body's well-being amid life's constant flux. As we delve deeper into its complexities, we develop a heightened admiration for the skin's resilience as it preserves the body's integrity among life's ever-changing circumstances.

The skin is one of the body's most adaptable organs, comprised of two primary layers: the epidermis and the dermis. Beneath the dermis lies the subcutaneous fascia, also known as the hypodermis. This layer, consisting of loose connective and adipose tissue, attaches to the skin and underlying organs; however, it is distinct from the skin itself (see Figure 1.1).

EPIDERMIS

The outermost layer of the skin is known as the epidermis. It is both superficial and thin, making it the most visible part of the skin. Although the skin envelops the entire body, there are notable regional differences that are associated with flexibility, hair distribution and type, gland density and type, pigmentation, vascularity, innervation and thickness. The thinnest section of skin, for example, is found on the eyelids. This measures just 0.5 mm in thickness, while the thickest aspect is found at the heel, where it reaches 4.0 mm. The epidermis is made up of epithelium called keratinised stratified squamous epithelium and contains four key cell types. These are:

1. Keratinocytes
2. Melanocytes
3. Langerhans cells
4. Merkel cells.

See Figure 1.2.

Keratinocytes   Arranged into four layers, these cells play a vital role in synthesising keratin, a durable, fibrous protein that is necessary for shielding the skin and underlying tissues from heat, microorganisms and chemicals. Additionally, the keratinocytes contribute to the skin's water-resistant qualities, serving as a protective barrier that minimises both water ingress and egress. Furthermore, these cells function as a sealant, preventing the infiltration of foreign substances.

Melanocytes   During embryonic development, melanocytes produce the pigment melanin, which contributes to the natural colouration of the skin. Melanocytes are most abundant in specific areas of the epidermis, such as the penis, nipples, areola, face and limbs. These cells feature elongated projections that interweave with keratinocytes, facilitating the transfer of melanin granules. Melanin serves a crucial role in shielding the skin from the harmful effects of sunlight.

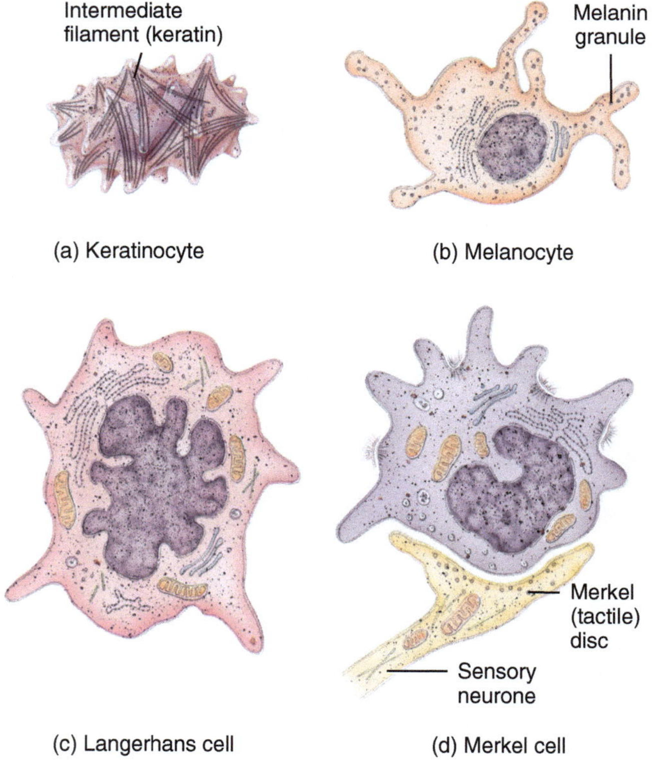

FIGURE 1.2   (a–d). The types of cells in the epidermis

Exposure to excessive sunlight prompts melanocytes to increase melanin production, absorbing more ultraviolet (UV) rays. Consequently, the skin darkens, resulting in a suntanned appearance – an indication of the skin's attempt to protect itself from damage. Although all individuals possess a similar number of melanocytes, those with brown or black skin produce more melanin, accounting for variations in skin colour. This increased melanin production and distribution provides greater natural protection against harmful UV radiation from the sun. Moles, also known as naevi, are clusters of melanocytes closely situated together. Figure 1.3 illustrates variations in skin colour and sensitivity to UV-induced burning.

Langerhans Cells   Langerhans cells are integral to the immune system, originating from the red bone marrow. After migrating from the bone marrow to the epidermis, they constitute a small portion of epidermal cells. These cells play a crucial role in regulating immune responses within the skin, serving as a defence against invading microorganisms. However, when exposed to sunlight, the Langerhans cells become delicate, impacting their function. Primarily, Langerhans cells are responsible for processing microbial antigens, which aids in stimulating lymphocytes. Their primary function is to support other immune cells in identifying and responding to microorganisms, ultimately facilitating the destruction of invading pathogens.

	Natural skin colour	UV sensitivity and tendency to burn
1	Very fair, pale white, often freckled	**Highly sensitive** Always burns, never tans
2	Fair, white skin	**Very sensitive** Burns easily, tans minimally
3	Light brown	**Sensitive** Burns moderately, usually tans
4	Moderate brown	**Less sensitive** Burns minimally tans well
5	Dark brown	**Minimally sensitive** Rarely burns
6	Deeply pigmented, dark brown to black	**Minimal sensitivity** Never burns

FIGURE 1.3   Skin colour and sensitivity to ultraviolet (UV)-induced burning

Merkel Cells Merkel cells possess the capacity to establish contact with a flattened process of a sensory neurone, forming a synaptic connection known as a tactile disc or Merkel disc. These Merkel cells, along with the tactile discs, are not very common in the epidermis but are highly skilled at detecting sensations of touch. These cells, along with the tactile discs, which are the least abundant cells in the epidermis, are adept at detecting sensations of touch.

LAYERS OF THE EPIDERMIS

Similar to the two distinct layers of skin, the dermis and epidermis, there are several other layers. These layers gradually form over time and comprise the epidermis. Known as strata, these layers are observable under a microscope (see Figure 1.4).

The superficial and deeper levels of the skin are:

- The stratum basale
- The stratum spinosum
- The stratum granulosum
- The stratum lucidum
- The stratum corneum.

Table 1.1 summarises the layers of the epidermis.

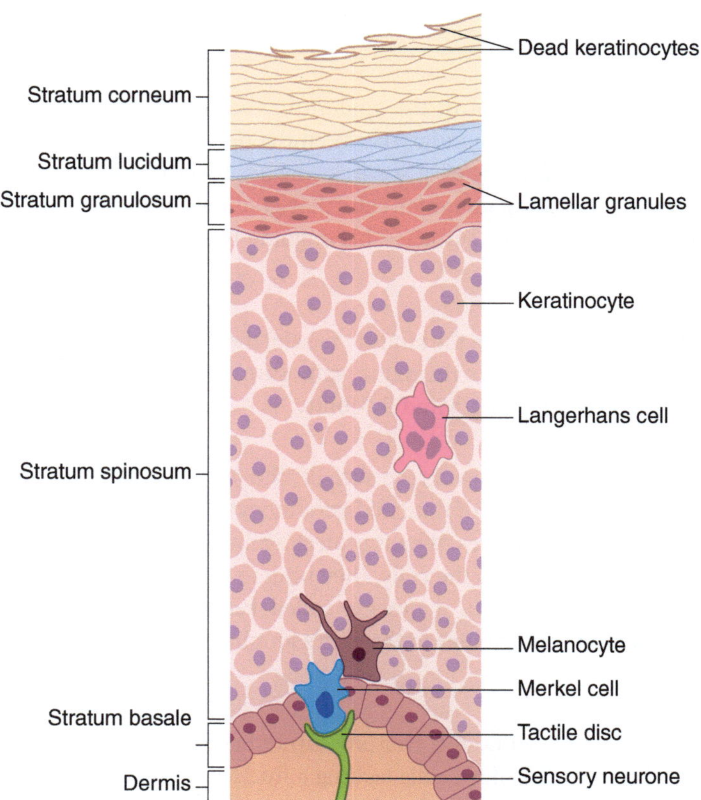

FIGURE 1.4 The layers of the epidermis

Table 1.1 Layers of the epidermis

Epidermal layer	Location	Description
Stratum basale (also known as the basal cell layer)	The deepest layer. It sits directly above the dermis.	Cuboidal cells arranged as a single row; these are constantly dividing and growing. The stratum basale also contains melanocytes and Merkel cells.
Stratum spinosum	Above the stratum basale and below the stratum granulosum.	These keratinocytes are tightly packed and flat and have spine-like projections.
Stratum granulosum	Under the stratum corneum.	Flattened cells arranged in around three to five layers. Protecting the body from losing fluid and from harm. Compact brittle cells as they lose their nucleus.
Stratum lucidum	When present, it is situated between the stratum corneum and the stratum granulosum.	These cells are not present on the soles and palms. The cells have no nucleus and are tightly packed.
Stratum corneum	The most superficial of layers.	Several layers of keratinised, dead epithelial cells. These cells are flattened and have no nucleus.

Stratum Basale The deepest layer of the epidermis, the stratum basale, rests upon the basement membrane, marking the boundary between the dermis and epidermis. Composed of a single row of columnar keratinocytes, it serves as the origin for new skin cells. These stem cells continually divide, generating daughter cells that gradually move upward through the epidermal layers until they reach the surface. This ongoing regeneration process ensures the skin's renewal.

Stratum Spinosum Situated above the stratum basale, the stratum spinosum houses keratinocytes with spiny projections, hence the name 'spinosum'. These keratinocytes are densely packed, providing the skin with strength and flexibility.

Stratum Granulosum Moving towards the surface, the next layer is the stratum granulosum, consisting of three to five layers of flattened keratinocytes. These cells contain granules, including water-resistant lipid granules, which protect against fluid loss and microbial invasion. As pressure from below flattens the cells, they undergo apoptosis, losing their nucleus and becoming compact and brittle in a process called keratinisation. This layer, located beneath the stratum lucidum, contributes to the skin's toughness and readiness for protective functions.

Stratum Lucidum Present below the stratum corneum, the stratum lucidum, or clear layer, consists of five layers of flat, dead cells lacking a nucleus. Found only in areas of thick skin, such as the heels, these tightly packed cells serve as a barrier to fluid loss.

Stratum Corneum The outermost layer of the epidermis, the stratum corneum, comprises approximately 25 layers of overlapping, scale-like dead cells predominantly made of keratin. With most of their fluid content lost, these tough, horny cells are covered in lipids, providing a protective barrier and structural strength. Continual friction leads to the shedding (sloughing off) of this layer, ensuring the skin's renewal.

DERMIS

The dermis, situated beneath the epidermis, constitutes the deepest layer of the skin. Primarily, it consists of dense connective tissue that is rich in collagen and elastic fibres, which houses a number of structures, including:

- Blood vessels
- Nerves
- Lymph vessels
- Smooth muscles
- Sweat glands
- Hair follicles
- Sebaceous glands

The elastic properties of the dermis offer support to the structures above it, which enables the skin to flex during movement and return to its original shape when at rest. Divided into two layers, the dermis comprises the papillary aspect and the reticular aspect. The papillary layers, resembling small projections, significantly increase the dermal surface area and anchor it to the epidermis, giving rise to fingerprints. Meanwhile, the deeper aspect of the dermis connects to the subcutaneous layer. Figure 1.5 illustrates the relationship between the epidermis, dermis and subcutaneous layer.

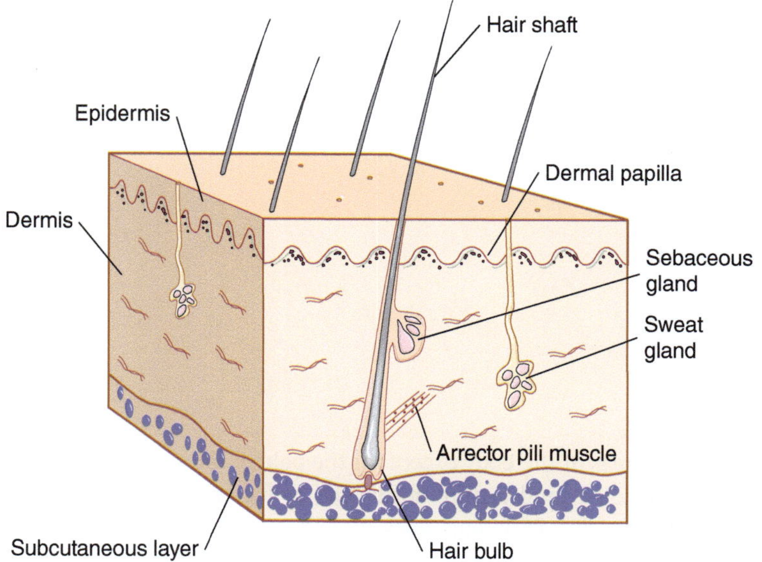

FIGURE 1.5 The epidermis, dermis and subcutaneous layer

Papillary and Reticular Aspects   The terms papillary aspect and reticular aspect refer to the two distinct layers or regions within the dermis, the deeper layer of the skin located beneath the epidermis. This is the superficial layer of the dermis characterised by finger-like projections known as papillae. These papillae extend upward and interlock with the epidermis, forming the boundary between the epidermis and dermis. The papillary aspect is responsible for the formation of ridges that are known as friction ridges, aiding in grip by increasing friction, particularly in the hands and feet.

Within the papillary aspect lies a network of capillaries and specialised sensory receptors known as Meissner's corpuscles, which respond to touch and temperature sensations. Nerve endings in this region are highly sensitive to various tactile stimuli, including warmth, coolness, pain and itching.

Attached to the subcutaneous layer, the reticular aspect comprises irregular, dense connective tissues containing fibroblasts, collagen bundles and coarse elastic fibres. The reticular aspect provides structural support and elasticity to the skin, allowing it to withstand stretching and deformation. This layer also contains additional sensory receptors, such as Pacinian receptors for deep sensory pressure. Furthermore, it accommodates accessory structures such as sweat glands, lymph vessels, smooth muscles and hair follicles.

THE SUBCUTANEOUS TISSUES

Subcutaneous tissues are also referred to as the subcutis or hypodermis, representing the deepest layer of the skin.

Comprising an essential protective barrier, the subcutaneous tissue consists of an insulating layer of fat and blood vessels. Its thickness varies across different body regions and among individuals. The fat within this layer serves to safeguard organs and bones, contributing to the regulation of body temperature by collaborating with blood vessels to maintain normal and consistent temperatures. Additionally, sweat glands in this layer play a vital role in thermoregulation. With advancing age, the subcutaneous tissue undergoes a natural thinning process.

ACCESSORY STRUCTURES OF THE SKIN

The accessory structures are also known as the appendages. The accessory structures of the skin include:

- Hair

- Skin glands

- Nails

HAIR

Hair is present on most areas of the body except for the palms, soles and lips, with variations in amount, distribution, colour and texture influenced by factors such as geographical location, gender, age and ethnicity. Different types of hair emerge during fetal development,

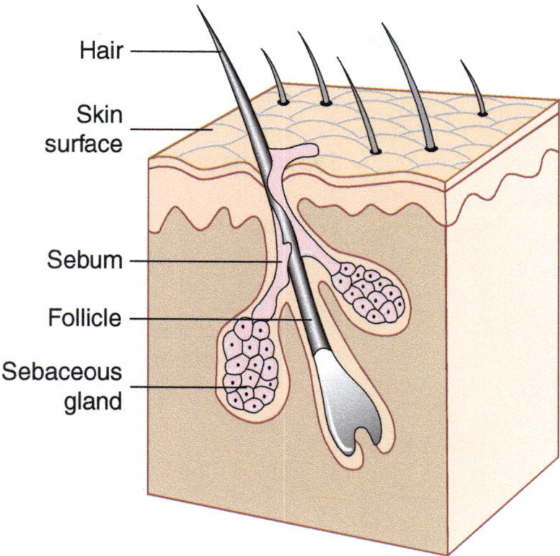

FIGURE 1.6 A pilosebaceous unit

starting with lanugo, a fine, non-pigmented downy hair that covers the fetus's body around the fifth month. Before birth, this lanugo is shed from areas such as the eyelashes, eyebrows and scalp, replaced by longer, coarser and pigmented hair (Brewster 2024).

Hair contributes to a person's distinctive appearance, with its colour influenced by melanocytes within the hair bulb. The greying of hair results from a progressive decline in melanin production, determined by genetic and hormonal factors.

Comprised of dead keratin, each hair is a thread that is formed from cells at the base of a follicle. Hair serves various functions, including sexual and social roles, thermoregulation and protection against external elements (Peate 2024). Primarily, hair acts to retain body heat, as hair follicles cover the entire skin surface, trapping heat between the hairs. The arrector pili muscles that are attached to each hair follicle contract in response to cold, fear or emotion, causing goosebumps on the skin.

Hair on the scalp shields the scalp from sun damage, while eyelashes and eyebrows protect the eyes from foreign particles and nose hair helps to prevent inhalation of foreign material. Sebaceous glands accompany hair follicles, secreting sebum, a liquid substance that lubricates the skin and hair, waterproofs them and removes waste. Sebum possesses antibacterial and antifungal properties, with the distribution of sebaceous glands being most prominent on the scalp, face, upper torso and anogenital region, particularly active during puberty due to hormonal influences. The base of the onion-shaped bulb – the follicle – contains blood vessels, providing nourishment for the developing hair. Figure 1.6 illustrates a pilosebaceous unit comprising the follicle, hair shaft, sebaceous gland and arrector pili muscle.

SKIN GLANDS

Within the skin, various glands act as miniature organs, serving multiple functions. Sweat glands (also known as sudoriferous glands), for instance, consist of coiled tubes that are composed of epithelial tissue that extends to pores on the skin surface (see Figure 1.7). Each gland has its own nerve and blood supply, producing a slightly acidic fluid containing water and salts. Sweat glands are classified into two types: eccrine and apocrine.

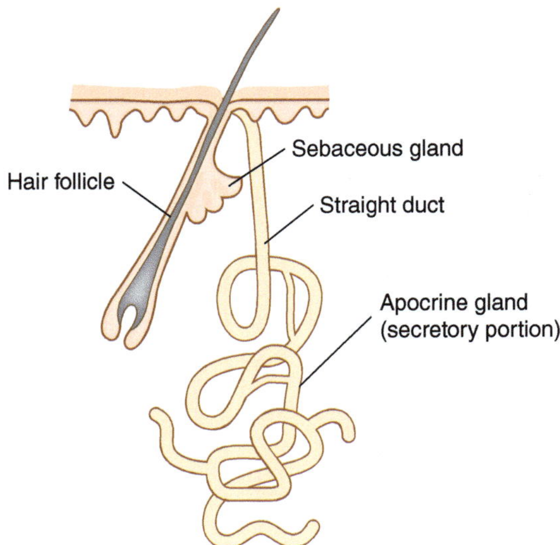

FIGURE 1.7   A sweat gland

ECCRINE GLANDS

The eccrine glands are primarily responsible for thermoregulation, which is the regulation of body temperature. They produce sweat, which is mainly composed of water and electrolytes. When the body becomes overheated, such as during physical activity, pyrexia or exposure to high temperatures, the eccrine glands release sweat onto the skin's surface. As this sweat evaporates, it helps to cool the body down, thus preventing overheating and maintaining a stable internal temperature. Additionally, eccrine sweat can also help to flush out toxins from the body and maintain hydration of the skin. These types of glands are located all over the body; however, there are sites where they are more numerous, such as the forehead, axillae, soles and palms.

APOCRINE GLANDS

The apocrine glands, like the eccrine glands, also have a coiled structure. However, they are less abundant and are localised in specific areas such as the pubic and axillary regions, nipples and perineum. The exact function of the apocrine glands is not fully understood; they become more active during puberty, producing thicker secretions than the eccrine glands, particularly during periods of stress or heightened emotions.

Several specialised types of apocrine glands exist. These include those that are located on the eyelids, the cerumen-producing glands found in the external auditory canal (ear wax glands) and also the milk-producing glands in the breasts.

Initially appearing on the palms and soles, apocrine glands gradually develop throughout the body. They are believed to secrete pheromones, which are released into the environment and communicate with others of the same species via olfaction, potentially eliciting sexual arousal reactions. When activated by surface bacteria, these glands secrete a viscous substance that results in body odour.

NAILS

The nails serve as a protective shield for the fingertips and toes. Composed of tightly packed, keratinised epidermal cells, they form a firm, solid layer over the digits (see Figure 1.8).

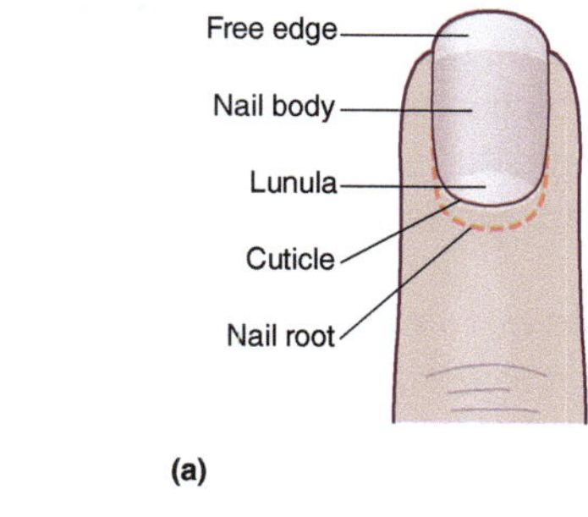

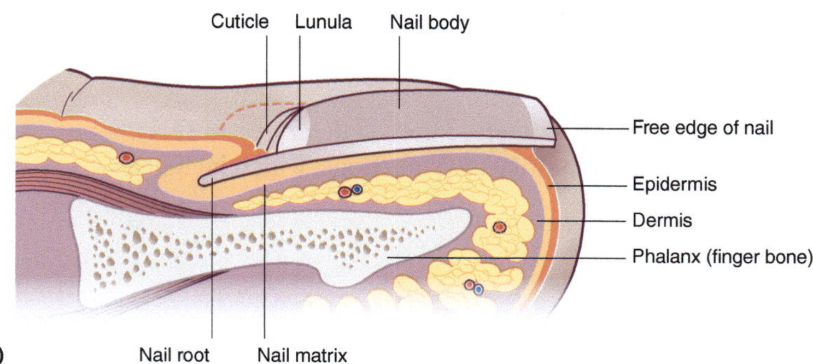

FIGURE 1.8   Nail

The horn-like structure of nails results from the concentrated keratin content. There are no nerve endings in nails. Nails serve as a tactile counterforce to fingertips, which are rich in nerve endings, enabling individuals to perceive sensations when objects are touched.

The pink hue of the nail body is due to underlying blood capillaries, while the white crescent-shaped area at the base, known as the lunula, results from air mixing with the keratin matrix. The size of the lunula varies among individuals. The cuticle, also called the eponychium, is a layer of stratum corneum extending over the proximal end of the nail body.

Fingernails grow faster than toenails, with nail growth slowing down as individuals age. On average, nails grow at a rate of 0.01 cm per day (equivalent to 1 cm per 100 days). It takes approximately four to six months for fingernails to completely regrow, while toenails require 12–18 months. Several factors, including age, season, level of physical activity and genetics, influence nail growth. Trauma, inflammation, injury or infection can delay nail growth and affect nail integrity. Additionally, systemic diseases such as chronic cardiopulmonary conditions or fungal infections can manifest through nail abnormalities.

ETHNICITY

Skin colour and ethnicity can influence various aspects of nail health and appearance.

Individuals with darker skin tones may have nails that appear darker due to increased melanin production in the nail matrix. Conversely, those with lighter skin tones may have nails with a lighter appearance. Additionally, certain ethnicities may exhibit unique nail characteristics, such as differences in lunula size or nail shape.

Nail growth rates can also vary depending on skin colour and ethnicity. People with darker skin tones may experience slower nail growth compared to those with lighter skin tones. This difference in growth rate may be attributed to variations in blood circulation and metabolism influenced by genetic factors and environmental conditions.

Furthermore, certain skin conditions, such as melanoma or psoriasis, may affect the appearance and health of the nails differently based on skin colour and ethnicity. For example, individuals with darker skin tones may be at a higher risk of developing subungual melanoma, a type of skin cancer that affects the nail unit, due to delayed diagnosis or misinterpretation of symptoms. See Mukwende, Tamony, and Turner (2020) for a handbook of clinical signs in black and brown skin.

Understanding these nuances can be important in clinical settings for accurately diagnosing and treating nail disorders, as well as for recognising potential indicators of systemic diseases that may manifest through nail abnormalities. It highlights the importance of considering skin colour and ethnicity as factors in assessing overall nail health and identifying any associated risks or concerns.

THE FUNCTIONS OF THE SKIN

A fundamental understanding of skin structure, as described in this chapter, can help the reader to begin to understand its multifaceted functions, which include:

- Sensation

- Thermoregulation

- Protection

- Excretion and absorption

- Synthesis of vitamin D

SENSATION

Located throughout the skin, there are numerous receptor sites that are capable of detecting changes in temperature and pressure in the surrounding environment. Comprising a diverse group of nerve endings, these receptors are distributed throughout the skin. Usually, the information that is gathered by these various receptors is relayed to the brain and the intricacies of sensory perception take place.

Sensations that originate in the skin are termed cutaneous sensations, while others include those that are related to vibration, tickling and irritation. Certain regions of the body boast a higher density of sensory receptors, such as the lips, genitalia and fingertips. Pain sensation may indicate either existing or potential tissue damage.

THERMOREGULATION

Thermoregulation is a vital function of the skin in maintaining homeostasis, ensuring that the body's temperature remains within narrow limits even during various activities. This process involves intricate adjustments to adapt to changes in external conditions. Effective thermoregulation is essential for survival, as temperature fluctuations can impact enzyme function and cellular composition.

The skin serves as a temperature regulator through a series of complex mechanisms. Modulation of blood vessel size in the skin is one such mechanism. When body temperature increases, blood vessels dilate (vasodilation), which facilitates the transfer of heat from deeper tissues to the skin's surface, where it can dissipate.

PROTECTION

The skin provides essential protection for the body through various mechanisms. For instance, melanin production shields against the harmful effects of UV light. Additionally, the skin maintains bodily integrity by accelerating cell turnover when necessary, shedding dead skin and facilitating cell migration, a key component of wound healing.

Through its network of over 2 million pores, the skin aids in eliminating waste products, thereby preventing the accumulation of toxins within the body. Moreover, it regulates fluid balance by controlling the secretion of sweat, preventing both dehydration and excessive fluid loss. Acting as a waterproof barrier, the skin also safeguards against harmful substances in the external environment from infiltrating the body. Sebum, excreted by the skin, contains antimicrobial compounds that can effectively eradicate surface bacteria. Additionally, the acidic pH of sweat production has the capacity to hinder bacterial growth. Within the dermis, phagocytic macrophages possess the capability to engulf and eliminate viruses and bacteria that have breached the skin's surface.

In Table 1.2, the skin's protective functions are explored further.

Table 1.2 The skin's protective functions

Protective function	Discussion
Barrier against pathogens	The skin serves as a physical barrier, preventing pathogens such as bacteria, viruses and fungi from entering the body. The outermost layer of the skin, the stratum corneum, is composed of tightly packed dead skin cells embedded in lipids, creating an impermeable barrier that microbes struggle to penetrate. Additionally, the slightly acidic pH of the skin's surface inhibits the growth of many microorganisms.
Immune response	Despite being a physical barrier, the skin is also an active participant in the body's immune response. Specialised immune cells, such as Langerhans cells and dendritic cells, patrol the skin, detecting and neutralising invading pathogens. These cells play a crucial role in initiating an immune response by presenting antigens to T cells, activating the body's adaptive immune system.
Sebum production	Sebaceous glands within the skin secrete an oily substance called sebum, which lubricates the skin and hair. Sebum contains antimicrobial properties that help prevent the growth of harmful bacteria on the skin's surface. By keeping the skin moisturised and creating a slightly acidic environment, sebum contributes to the skin's overall defence against pathogens.
Regulation of pH	The skin maintains a slightly acidic pH, typically ranging from 4.5 to 5.5. This acidic environment inhibits the growth of many harmful microorganisms while promoting the growth of beneficial bacteria that help protect against pathogens. Disruptions in the skin's pH balance can compromise its protective function and increase susceptibility to infections.
Physical protection	Beyond its role in immune defence, the skin provides physical protection against environmental hazards such as UV radiation, extreme temperatures and mechanical injuries. The epidermis, dermis and subcutaneous tissue work together to absorb and distribute impact forces, reducing the risk of tissue damage from bumps, falls or other traumatic events.
Sensory protection	Sensory receptors in the skin provide feedback to the central nervous system, alerting the body to potential threats or hazards in the environment. Pain receptors, for example, signal tissue damage, prompting protective responses such as reflex withdrawal or behavioural avoidance.

The skin's protective functions encompass a sophisticated collection of physical, chemical and immunological mechanisms that work together to safeguard the body from external threats and maintain its overall health and integrity.

EXCRETION AND ABSORPTION

The skin possesses the capacity to eliminate substances from the body; sweat, for instance, comprises water, sodium, carbon dioxide, ammonia and urea. Jenkins and Tortora (2016) highlight that despite its nearly impermeable nature, the body can excrete around 400 mL of water daily. Individuals leading sedentary lifestyles typically excrete less, whereas those engaged in more active pursuits excrete more.

Moreover, the skin serves as a conduit for absorption from the external environment. Various materials are absorbed into body cells from the surroundings, some of which, upon absorption, can pose toxicity risks, such as heavy metals, for example, lead and mercury. Additionally, certain therapeutic and non-therapeutic medications can be absorbed through the skin. Notably, fat-soluble vitamins A, D, E and K, as well as oxygen and carbon dioxide, are among the substances that can be absorbed through the skin.

SYNTHESIS OF VITAMIN D

The skin plays an active role in synthesising vitamin D. Sunlight triggers a process in the skin that produces vitamin D, a vital nutrient for bone health and overall well-being. This process begins when sunlight activates a molecule in the skin, leading to the formation of vitamin D. The newly formed vitamin D then undergoes transformations in the liver and kidneys, ultimately converting into its active form, known as calcitriol (a hormone). Calcitriol plays a crucial role in facilitating the absorption of calcium from the diet, essential for maintaining bone strength, muscle function and overall health. Insufficient levels of calcitriol can lead to weakened bones and increased susceptibility to various health issues. Therefore, ensuring adequate exposure to sunlight and consuming foods rich in vitamin D are important for maintaining optimal health.

CONCLUSION

The anatomy and physiology of the skin extends beyond its structural intricacies to encompass its dynamic interactions with the body's internal systems and external environment. Beyond its protective barrier function, the skin serves as a sensory interface that conveys tactile sensations, temperature changes and emotional responses. Its role in thermoregulation ensures the maintenance of optimal body temperature, while its vascular network facilitates nutrient exchange and waste removal.

Additionally, the skin's immune surveillance mechanisms act as vigilant defenders against invading microbes and harmful pathogens, highlighting its essential role in the body's defence system. The skin's ability to synthesise vitamin D underlines its metabolic significance, influencing calcium homeostasis, bone health and immune function.

In the field of pathology, the skin reveals a diverse range of conditions, from benign dermatological disorders to life-threatening diseases. Understanding the underlying pathophysiology of skin conditions enables those who offer care and support to diagnose, treat and manage these conditions effectively.

GLOSSARY OF TERMS

Apocrine glands: Sweat glands found in areas such as the axillary and pubic regions, activated during emotional stress and puberty.

Basal layer: Also known as the stratum basale, the deepest layer of the epidermis where new skin cells are produced.

Collagen: A protein present in the dermis that provides structural support and elasticity to the skin.

Dermis: The middle layer of the skin containing blood vessels, nerves, sweat glands and hair follicles.

Epidermis: The outermost layer of the skin responsible for providing waterproofing and protecting against external threats.

Follicle: The structure surrounding the root of a hair strand within the skin.

Keratin: A protein found in the epidermis that provides strength and waterproofing to the skin.

Hypodermis: Also known as the subcutaneous layer, it consists of fat and connective tissue that insulates the body and anchors the skin to underlying structures.

Immune system: The body's defence mechanism against pathogens and foreign invaders, including those affecting the skin.

Keratinocytes: Cells found in the epidermis responsible for producing keratin, the primary structural protein of the skin.

Langerhans cells: Specialised immune cells found in the epidermis that help protect against pathogens.

Melanin: A pigment produced by melanocytes in the epidermis that gives skin its colour and provides protection against ultraviolet (UV) radiation.

Sebaceous glands: Glands in the skin that produce sebum, an oily substance that lubricates and protects the skin and hair.

Sweat glands: Eccrine glands in the skin that produce sweat, helping to regulate body temperature and excrete waste products.

Thermoregulation: The process by which the body maintains a stable internal temperature through mechanisms such as sweating and shivering.

UV radiation: Invisible rays from the sun that can damage the skin and increase the risk of skin cancer.

Vitamin D: A nutrient synthesised by the skin in response to sunlight exposure, essential for calcium absorption and bone health.

MULTIPLE CHOICE QUESTIONS

1. What is the outermost layer of the skin called?
   a) Dermis
   b) Epidermis
   c) Hypodermis
   d) Basal layer

2. Which pigment is responsible for giving colour to the skin?
   a) Melatonin
   b) Haemoglobin
   c) Melanin
   d) Keratin

3. Which layer of the skin contains blood vessels, nerves and hair follicles?
   a) Epidermis
   b) Dermis
   c) Hypodermis
   d) Basal layer

4. What is the primary function of sebaceous glands?
   a) Producing sweat
   b) Regulating body temperature
   c) Producing sebum to lubricate the skin and hair
   d) Secreting melanin

5. Which type of sweat glands are responsible for regulating body temperature?
   a) Eccrine glands
   b) Apocrine glands
   c) Sebaceous glands
   d) Ceruminous glands

6. What is the primary protein found in the skin, hair and nails?
   a) Collagen
   b) Elastin
   c) Keratin
   d) Melanin

7. What type of cells are responsible for producing new skin cells in the epidermis?
   a) Melanocytes
   b) Keratinocytes
   c) Langerhans cells
   d) Merkel cells

8. What is the function of Langerhans cells in the epidermis?
   a) Producing melanin pigment
   b) Detecting deep pressure and vibration
   c) Regulating body temperature
   d) Acting as immune cells against pathogens

9. What is the primary function of hair on the body?
   a) Detecting touch sensations
   b) Regulating body temperature
   c) Protecting against UV radiation
   d) Providing insulation and sensation

10. What is the main function of the arrector pili muscles associated with hair follicles?
    a) Regulating body temperature
    b) Contracting to produce goosebumps
    c) Producing sebum to lubricate the skin
    d) Stimulating melanocytes to produce melanin

REFERENCES

Brewster, J. (2024). Embryology and fetal development (Chapter 4). In: *Fundamentals of Maternal Anatomy and Physiology* (eds. I. Peate and C. Leader). Oxford: Wiley.

Evans, S. (2022). Basic scientific principles of physiology (Chapter 1). In: *Fundamentals of Anatomy and Physiology*, 3e (eds. I. Peate and S. Evans). Oxford: Wiley.

Jenkins, G.W. and Tortora, G.J. (2016). *Anatomy and Physiology*. New Jersey: Wiley.

McLaughlin, M.F. (2018). Integumentary issues (Chapter 4). In: *Perianesthesia Nursing Care*, 2e (eds. D. Stannard and D.A. Krenzischek). Burlington: Jones and Bartlett.

Mukwende, M., Tamony, P. and Turner, M. (2020). *Mind the Gap: A Handbook of Clinical Signs in Black and Brown Skin* London: St George's, University of London.

Peate, I. (2019). *Fundamentals of Assessment and Care Planning for Nurses*. Oxford: Wiley.

Peate, I. (2020). The skin (Chapter 18). In: *Fundamentals of Anatomy and Physiology*, 3e (eds. I. Peate and S. Evans). Oxford: Wiley.

Peate, I. (2024). Men and hair loss: A guide for primary care nurse. *Independent Nurse* 2024 (5): 22–25.

Stephens, M. (2021). The skin and associated disorder (Chapter 20). In: *Fundamentals of Applied Pathophysiology*, 4e (ed. I. Peate). Oxford: Wiley.

Effective skin assessment involves a multifaceted approach that begins with education. This requires those who offer care and support to have an understanding of the intricacies of skin anatomy and physiology (see Chapter 1 of this book), understanding the normal characteristics of healthy skin, such as its colour, temperature, moisture, texture and turgor. Developing insight into common skin conditions, including their causes, symptoms and treatments, will establish a strong grounding for enhancing assessment skills. It is important to have a good understanding of various skin conditions as they are often complex with numerous possible diagnoses (McPhillips et al. 2021). With this knowledge, those who offer care and support to people can confidently engage with patients regarding their skin health and related issues.

Once equipped with knowledge, it is essential to refine observation skills. Practice systematically observing the skin, ensuring careful attention is paid to even the slightest changes in colour, texture and overall condition. Be observant for signs of inflammation, lesions or discolouration, as these can be indicative of underlying issues requiring attention.

The next step involves acquiring assessment techniques and gaining proficiency in various methods, including inspection and palpation. It can take time to perfect these skills. Understanding how to use standardised assessment tools and scales is essential for effectively assessing pressure ulcer risk. Practicing assessments on different body areas, particularly those prone to pressure injuries, is crucial for ensuring thorough and accurate evaluations.

Documentation is a crucial aspect of skin assessment. Documenting findings accurately and comprehensively, using a standardised approach that includes detailed descriptions of any abnormalities, their location, size and associated symptoms is essential. Clear and concise communication through documentation is essential for effective continuity of care. Local policy and procedure must be adhered to at all times.

Seeking guidance from experienced health care professionals, clinical educators and others is invaluable. Take advantage of clinical opportunities to practice skin assessment under supervision, actively seeking feedback and incorporating any feedback or suggestions into your practice. Use resources such as textbooks, online materials and educational resources to expand knowledge and stay updated on evidence-based practices in skin care.

Continuous improvement is key. Recognise that skin assessment is a skill that requires ongoing practice and refinement. Seek out opportunities for professional development through workshops, continuing education courses and self-directed learning. Reflect on your practice regularly, identifying areas for improvement and setting goals for further development based on feedback from peers, mentors and patients.

Approach skin assessment with empathy, respect and compassion. Bear in mind that each assessment activity represents an opportunity to provide patient-centred care. Ensuring the comfort and dignity of patients, building trust and involving them in the assessment process whenever possible are prioritised.

Embracing a lifelong learning mindset and staying committed to excellence, can help to develop and improve the provision of skilled and compassionate skin care in a range of health and care environments.

ASSESSING THE SKIN

Skin assessment (this may also include hair and nails) is a critical aspect of care provision, as the skin serves as a window into a patient's overall health. By examining the skin, valuable information about a patient's medical history, current condition and potential underlying issues can be gathered.

When conducting a skin assessment, both subjective and objective data are collected. Subjective data is obtained through patient interviews and discussions, where patients may describe symptoms, concerns or previous skin conditions. Objective data, on the other hand, is collected through direct observation and physical examination of the skin. See Table 2.1 gathering subjective and objective data to obtain a comprehensive understanding of the patient's skin health.

Table 2.1   Subjective and objective data – assessing the skin

Subjective data	Objective data
Refers to information provided by the patient through interviews or discussions, which includes the patient's own perceptions, experiences and descriptions of their skin condition.	Involves information gathered through direct observation and physical examination of the skin.
Symptoms:	Skin inspection:
Patients may report symptoms such as itching, pain, burning or discomfort in specific areas of the skin. These symptoms can provide valuable insight into the nature and severity of the skin problem.	The skin is visually inspected for abnormalities, lesions, rashes, discolouration or any other visible changes. The colour, texture, moisture and overall integrity of the skin are assessed.
Patient history:	Palpation:
Patients may provide information about their past medical history, including any previous skin conditions, allergies or surgery. Understanding the patient's medical background helps assess risk factors and tailor interventions accordingly.	The hands are used to palpate or touch the skin to assess for temperature, texture, turgor and any areas of tenderness or swelling. Palpation helps identify subtle abnormalities that may not be apparent during visual inspection alone.
Medications and treatment:	Measurement:
Patients may disclose any medications they are currently taking, including topical creams, ointments or oral medications prescribed for skin conditions. They may also discuss previous treatments or remedies they have tried for their skin issues.	The size, shape and location of specific skin lesions or wounds are measured using standardised techniques and tools. Measurements provide objective data for tracking changes in the skin over time and evaluating the effectiveness of interventions.
Lifestyle factors:	Documentation:
Patients may share details about their daily routines, habits and environmental exposures that could impact skin health. This may include factors such as occupation, hobbies, skincare practices, sun exposure and use of cosmetics or skincare products.	Findings are accurately and comprehensively documented, recording details such as the location, size, colour, shape and characteristics of any abnormalities observed. Clear and concise documentation is essential for communication with other healthcare providers and continuity of care. Local policies and procedures are followed regarding standards for documentation.

The importance of taking a comprehensive history during skin assessments has been emphasised by Bickley, Szilagyi, and Hoffman (2024). This involves asking detailed questions about the patient's skin concerns, past medical history, medications, allergies and lifestyle factors that may impact skin health. Additionally, specific questions related to the current skin problem, such as onset, duration, aggravating factors and associated symptoms, are essential for accurate assessment and diagnosis.

In addition to obtaining a thorough history, a systematic physical examination of the skin is essential. This includes inspecting the skin for colour, texture, moisture, temperature and turgor. The skin is gently palpated to assess for any abnormalities, such as lumps, lesions or areas of tenderness. Systematically assessing the entire body can help identify any areas of concern and monitor changes over time.

The skin is unique in that it is not only easily accessible for examination, but it also serves as a barrier between the body and the external environment. As a result, it is more susceptible to injury, infection and other adverse effects. During assessing of the skin, vigilance is needed to observe for signs of injury, such as cuts, bruises or abrasions, as well as signs of infection, for example, redness, swelling or discharge.

Furthermore, the skin can provide valuable clues about underlying health conditions. For example, jaundice, a yellowing of the skin and eyes, may indicate liver dysfunction, while cyanosis, a bluish discolouration of the skin, may indicate poor oxygenation. By recognising these signs and symptoms, appropriate interventions can be initiated and collaboration with other healthcare providers undertaken to ensure optimum patient care.

VARIATIONS IN PRESENTATIONS BETWEEN DARK AND LIGHT SKIN

Understanding the variations in dermatological presentations between individuals with dark and light skin is essential for providing safe and effective care that meets the specific needs of patients with diverse skin tones.

PIGMENTATION DIFFERENCES

Dark skin contains more melanin, which can affect the appearance of skin conditions. For example, inflammatory conditions such as eczema may appear darker or hyperpigmented in dark skin, making them more challenging to diagnose compared to their presentation in light skin. An awareness of these differences is required to accurately assess and manage skin conditions in those patients with dark skin.

HAIR TYPES

Dark skin is often associated with coarser hair types, which can influence the development and presentation of skin conditions. Conditions such as folliculitis or ingrown hair may be more prevalent in individuals with coarse hair, requiring tailored treatment approaches.

NORMAL CHANGES IN DARK SKIN

Understanding the normal variations in dark skin is key for distinguishing between benign changes and potential pathology. For instance, post-inflammatory hyperpigmentation, commonly seen after resolving skin conditions such as acne or eczema, may appear more pronounced in dark skin. There is a need to differentiate between normal variations and signs of underlying disease to avoid unnecessary interventions.

CHANGES IN COLOUR AND PRESENTATION

Skin conditions may present differently in dark skin compared to light skin. For example, conditions such as vitiligo or psoriasis may have distinct presentations in dark skin, requiring careful observation and assessment. Additionally, certain conditions, such as keloids or hypertrophic scars, may be more prevalent in individuals with dark skin and require specialised management strategies.

Understanding these nuances can help with the provision of culturally sensitive and effective care to patients with dark skin. This includes conducting thorough skin assessments, recognising variations in presentation and implementing tailored treatment plans that consider the unique characteristics of those with a darker skin. Additionally, it is important to engage with ongoing education and training to help stay updated on best practice for caring for patients with diverse skin types.

Mind the Gap: A Handbook of Clinical Signs in Black and Brown Skin (Mukwende et al. 2020) is a handbook designed to address the gap in medical education regarding the recognition and diagnosis of skin conditions in individuals with darker skin tones. The title 'Mind the Gap' alludes to the need to bridge the gap in knowledge and awareness of skin presentations in diverse populations. This handbook provides essential information to help accurately identify and treat skin conditions in patients with black and brown skin. It includes descriptions and images related to skin conditions in individuals with darker skin tones. The overall aim is to improve healthcare outcomes and reduce disparities in skin care.

Skin assessment is a fundamental component of practice that requires a comprehensive approach. By obtaining a detailed history, performing a thorough physical examination and interpreting findings accurately, this can help to identify skin problems, monitor changes over time and promote skin health and overall well-being.

THE PATIENT HISTORY

Obtaining a thorough understanding of the patient's overall health history is crucial for making a definitive diagnosis. By exploring the patient's skin history, valuable information about the patient's main complaints and any underlying local or systemic health problems that may be contributing to their skin issues may be identified.

The most frequent skin complaints typically include itching, various types of skin lesions (such as nodules) and rashes (Bickley, Szilagyi, and Hoffman 2024; Tidman 2018). Chief complaints may also involve changes in existing lesions and hair loss.

Gathering details about the current illness requires inquiring about lesions and rashes. Questions about onset (initial appearance) and duration, whether there are solitary or multiple lesions and their specific locations are essential. Patients should describe the size, shape, elevation and colour of the lesions. Additionally, the presence of crusting, exudate or pain should be noted. At this point in the consultation, the person offering care and support may request to visually inspect the lesions or rash. It is important to determine if there are any alterations in size, shape, elevation and colour since onset. Assessing if there are accompanying symptoms such as fever, itching, pain, headaches or other systemic disturbances is also key.

EXUDATE

Exudate refers to fluid that oozes out of tissues or blood vessels as a result of inflammation or injury. It typically contains proteins, inflammatory cells and tissue debris. Exudate plays a crucial role in the body's healing process by helping to remove dead cells and debris from the site of injury and providing nutrients and growth factors to support tissue repair. However, excessive or abnormal exudate production can impede wound healing and may indicate underlying issues such as infection or poor circulation. Exudate is commonly observed in wounds, ulcers and inflammatory conditions.

Assessment of exudate is based on its colour, consistency, odour and volume. Typically, it appears clear, amber-coloured and odourless. Exudate should be described and documented related to the colour and consistency of the fluid (see Box 2.1). A simpler way to gauge volume is by examining how the dressing interacts after use: is it dry, moist, wet, saturated or leaking? This method aids in determining whether exudate levels have increased, decreased or remained unchanged.

BOX 2.1 EXUDATE

- Serous (clear) or straw-coloured exudate: usually considered normal; however, if not clear and watery, it may indicate infection.
- Fibrinous exudate: appears cloudy and thin, containing fibrin protein strands; considered normal.
- Serosanguinous exudate: exhibits a clear, pink and watery appearance; generally normal.
- Sanguineous exudate: appears red, thin and watery, indicating trauma to blood vessels.
- Seropurulent exudate: appears murky or yellow, with a thick and creamy texture, suggesting active infection.
- Purulent exudate: appears yellow, grey or green, with a thick consistency, indicating infection.
- Haemopurulent exudate: appears dark, blood-stained, viscous and sticky, containing neutrophils, dead/dying bacteria and inflammatory cells, indicating an established infection. Damage to dermal capillaries leads to blood leakage.
- Haemorrhagic exudate: appears red, thick and usually infected, caused by trauma. Capillaries easily break down; this leads to spontaneous bleeding. It should not be confused with bloody exudate resulting from excessive debridement.

Source: Adapted from Stephens (2022); World Union of Wound Healing Societies (2019).

The patient is asked if there have been any instances of prior skin trauma, malignancy, exposure to chemicals or irritants. Has the patient recently consumed any new foods? Additionally, what medications are the patient currently taking? These factors are known as precipitating factors.

The patient may describe what exacerbates the primary complaint. They may also provide details about factors that alleviate the complaint, which could include over-the-counter or prescribed medications.

The patient's medical history is just as essential for skin assessments, as it is for other health conditions. Information obtained during this stage can reveal recurrences, flare-ups, triggers or patterns associated with the condition.

PAST SURGERY

Has the individual undergone any recent surgical procedures? Surgery disrupts the skin's natural defences, which can potentially lead to inflammation and infection. Conditions such as immunodeficiency, endocrine disorders and thromboembolism may influence skin treatment.

SKIN, NAIL AND HAIR CONDITION

Has there been a history of skin cancer? Are there any existing nail or hair conditions and if so, what treatments have been used?

SUNLIGHT SENSITIVITY

Individuals who are intolerant to sunlight are at a heightened risk of developing skin cancer. Has the person experienced any episodes of sunburn in the past?

ALLERGY ASSESSMENT

Does the individual have any known allergies? Have they undergone any allergy testing and if so, do they know what the outcome was?

FAMILY AND SOCIAL HISTORY

Family and social history are important aspects to consider in skin assessments. Many skin disorders have familial or genetic components. Therefore, it is crucial to explore the patient's family history, gathering information about parents, siblings, causes of death in the family and any chronic diseases or skin disorders.

Social history provides additional insights. The patient's occupation, for example, can influence their risk of skin cancer, especially if it involves prolonged sun exposure. Occupations involving chemical contact or exposure to latex gloves may increase the risk of contact dermatitis, so these factors should be noted and reported. Asking about hobbies and potential exposure to chemicals is also important.

Inquiring about smoking habits is essential, as smoking can suppress the immune system and hinder the body's ability to repair cell damage. Similarly, alcohol consumption should be assessed to understand its potential impact on skin health. Recreational use of amphetamines can lead to skin-related problems such as dry, itchy skin. Additionally, asking about foreign travel helps to consider the risk of tropical infections. When asking patients about a skin condition in relation to hair and nails, questions noted in Table 2.2 may be considered.

Table 2.2   Assessment of the hair and nails

Hair	Are there any recent changes in hair appearance or texture?
	Have you noticed increased hair loss, thinning or bald patches?
	Has there been a change in the distribution of hair across your body?
	Have you recently started using different hair products?
	Have you recently started a new diet?
	Have you observed any unusual increase in hair growth (hirsutism) and if so, where?
Nails	Have there been any recent alterations in nail appearance?
	Do you notice any splitting, breakage or changes in colour?
	Are there any visible indications of infection?
	Have there been recent dietary changes, dieting practices or exposure to chemicals?

Source: Adapted from Stephens (2022).

PHYSICAL EXAMINATION

Following the collection of subjective data, a physical examination is performed to gain a comprehensive understanding of the patient and their skin condition. Mukwende et al. (2020) proposes that the skin examination is made up of a general assessment as well as a specific skin assessment, which may be part of a comprehensive evaluation or a targeted assessment for those individuals with known or suspected issues.

The environment in which the examination is to be conducted must be given careful consideration, as the patient may need to disrobe. It is essential to provide a clear explanation for this requirement. The examination area should be well-lit with natural light, private and comfortably warm. Curtains should be drawn for privacy and the patient should wear a gown to preserve dignity and prevent unnecessary exposure of unaffected body areas. Depending on the location of the skin disorder, the patient may be examined while standing, sitting or lying down. Those offering care and support to the patient may need to assist them into these positions, as well as provide clear instructions.

Personal protective equipment should be worn when examining open lesions, infections, infestations or oozing wounds or mucous membranes, following local policies and procedures. Some lesions may require measurement or photography, while others necessitate close visual inspection.

Equipment needed for the physical examination includes:

- Gloves
- A good light source
- Magnification tool
- Clear ruler
- Measuring grids
- Tape measures
- Camera and photography consent forms

(Bickley, Szilagyi, and Hoffman 2024).

INSPECTION

There may have been some aspects of observation that may have occurred during the health interview (history taking). The condition of the skin often provides insights into the patient's overall health status, reflecting their self-care abilities and mental and emotional well-being.

A fundamental component of the physical assessment involves tactile examination of the patient and their skin. It is imperative to obtain the patient's consent before proceeding. The examination should ideally take place in a clinical setting with ample natural lighting. Initially, the patient may feel embarrassed or uncomfortable. This emphasises the importance of establishing a therapeutic relationship and offering to provide a chaperone. The outcome of this must be documented.

The ability to touch the skin provides valuable information about the patient and their skin condition. Various aspects are assessed, including the skin's colour in relation to ethnicity and also the chief complaint; note its texture, temperature, moisture level, turgor and the presence of oedema. Additionally, other findings may be observed, such as scars, missing digits or limbs and any open wounds. Lesions are evaluated for their distribution, characteristics and shape, along with noting their site and location, as outlined in Table 2.3.

When documenting skin findings, it is essential to ensure that detailed and precise descriptions of observed characteristics are noted. Notes should include details about the size, shape, arrangement, colour, texture, elevation, depression and presence of pedunculation (with or without a stalk). It should be noted that secondary lesions may overlay primary ones, which can potentially obscure identification and may require magnification for clarification. See Figures 2.1 and 2.2 for primary lesion terminology and secondary lesion terminology.

Table 2.3   Characteristics, distribution and shape of lesions

Characteristics	Shape	Distribution
Is there any redness, scaling, crusting or exudate observed? Are there any excoriations, blisters, erosions, pustules or papules present? Do the lesions appear uniform (monomorphic), resembling a drug rash, or do they vary (polymorphic), as seen in conditions such as chickenpox?	Are the lesions of varying sizes (small, large) and shapes such as circular or linear? Do they exhibit distinct borders? Are they flat or fluid-filled? Is there any induration present?	Observe if the condition is present on the hands, feet, extremities, ears and nose, particularly in areas exposed to light, or is it predominantly confined to the trunk? Is the distribution of the condition localised or widespread? If it is widespread, is the presentation symmetrical and is it centrally or peripherally located? Does the condition appear linear, regional (e.g. in the groin) or does it follow a dermatomal pattern such as shingles?

Source: Adapted from Stephens (2022), Peters (2019), and Bickley, Szilagyi, and Hoffman (2024).

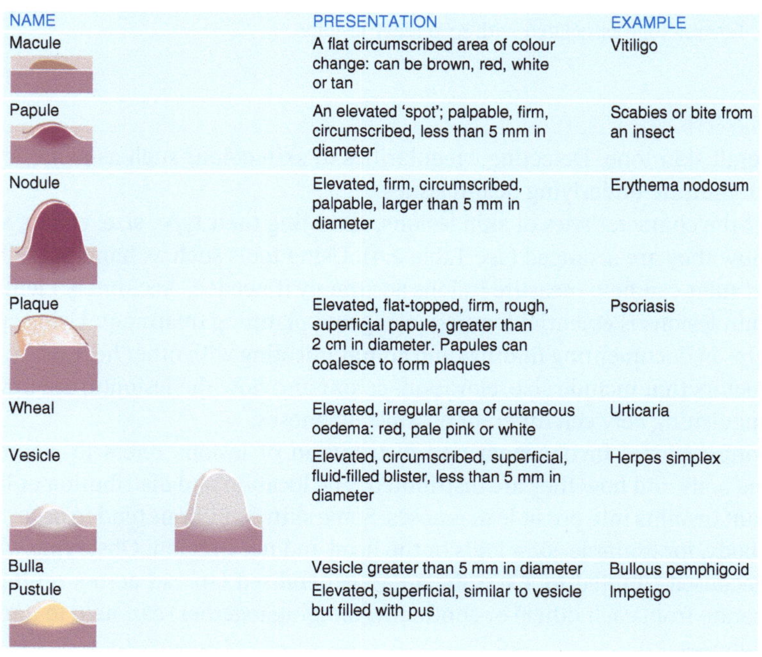

NAME	PRESENTATION	EXAMPLE
Macule	A flat circumscribed area of colour change: can be brown, red, white or tan	Vitiligo
Papule	An elevated 'spot'; palpable, firm, circumscribed, less than 5 mm in diameter	Scabies or bite from an insect
Nodule	Elevated, firm, circumscribed, palpable, larger than 5 mm in diameter	Erythema nodosum
Plaque	Elevated, flat-topped, firm, rough, superficial papule, greater than 2 cm in diameter. Papules can coalesce to form plaques	Psoriasis
Wheal	Elevated, irregular area of cutaneous oedema: red, pale pink or white	Urticaria
Vesicle	Elevated, circumscribed, superficial, fluid-filled blister, less than 5 mm in diameter	Herpes simplex
Bulla	Vesicle greater than 5 mm in diameter	Bullous pemphigoid
Pustule	Elevated, superficial, similar to vesicle but filled with pus	Impetigo

FIGURE 2.1   Terminology associated with primary lesions

NAME	PRESENTATION	EXAMPLE
Scale	Thickened, flaky exfoliation, irregular, thick or thin, dry or oily, variable size, silver, white or tan in colour	Psoriasis
Crust	Dried serum, blood or purulent exudate; slightly elevated; size variable	Impetigo discoid
Excoriation	Loss of epidermis caused by scratching	Atopic eczema
Lichenification	Rough thickened epidermis, accentuated skin markings due to scratching	Lichen simplex

FIGURE 2.2   Terminology associated with secondary lesions

SKIN EXAMINATION

Examine overall skin tone. Detecting irregularities in skin colour such as pallor, cyanosis or erythema can indicate underlying health issues.

Inspect the characteristics of skin lesions, including their type, size, colour, shape, elevation and how they are arranged (see Table 2.4). Using tools such as hand magnification or a transparent ruler can help measure lesions accurately if needed. Accurately identifying and classifying skin lesions is essential for diagnosing and planning treatment. Using specific terminology helps in documenting findings and communicating with other healthcare providers. Evaluating factors that include size, elevation, colour and how the lesion(s) are arranged can help in distinguishing between different possible diagnoses.

Assessing regional involvement and distribution of lesions refers to where they are located on the body and how they are distributed. The location and distribution of lesions can offer important insights into possible diagnoses. Some skin conditions tend to occur in specific areas of the body, for example, skin folds or the head and neck region. Observing whether the lesions are localised (limited to a specific area), generalised (spread across multiple areas), discrete (separate from each other) or confluent (merging together) can help to narrow down potential diagnoses.

Table 2.4   Lesions, terminology

A lesion refers to any individual area of altered skin, which may occur as solitary or multiple. A rash refers to a widespread outbreak of lesions. Dermatosis is the term that is used to describe a skin disease.	
Granuloma	A mass of immune cells that forms in response to infection, inflammation or foreign substances.
Fungating	Refers to the rapid growth of a tumour or lesion that protrudes from the skin surface.
Excoriation	A superficial injury to the skin caused by scratching or abrasion.
Exudate	Fluid that oozes out of tissue due to inflammation or injury, often seen as pus or serum.
Lichenification	Thickening and hardening of the skin, usually due to chronic irritation or scratching.
Psoriasiform	Resembling the appearance of psoriasis, a chronic inflammatory skin condition characterised by red, scaly patches.
Vesicle	A small fluid-filled blister on the skin, usually less than 5 mm in diameter.
Bulla	A larger fluid-filled blister on the skin, typically greater than 5 mm in diameter.
Plaque	A raised, flat-topped lesion on the skin, often associated with scaling or inflammation.
Sessile	Referring to a growth or lesion that is attached directly to the skin surface without a stalk or stem.

Source: Adapted from Rhoads and Wiggins Petersen (2021).

HAIR AND NAIL ASSESSMENT

After examining the skin, the hair and nails are then assessed. To begin, the patient's hair is inspected, with an explanation provided for the examination. Note the colour, texture and distribution of the hair, while also observing for any signs of scale or erythema on the scalp. Excessive hair growth in females, known as hirsutism, may occur in areas typically associated with male hair growth, such as the beard, moustache, upper back, shoulders, sternum, axillae and pubic region. Hirsutism can be indicative of endocrine disorders or may have an unknown cause (idiopathic). Additionally, alopecia areata, an autoimmune disorder that is characterised by hair loss in round patches, should be noted as a potential concern. Alopecia totalis refers to the complete loss of scalp hair, while alopecia universalis involves total hair loss across the entire body.

The patient's nails are examined next, noting their consistency, texture and any separation of the nail plate from the nail bed. Healthy nails should have a smooth, consistent surface, and signs of fungal infection should be observed. The nails should be translucent in colour, changes in colour may indicate infection. Additionally, a capillary refill test is performed, and the results are recorded.

Visual inspection is a vital assessment technique, providing valuable information about the patient's skin. Palpation can further aid in diagnosis, although gloves should be used whenever there is open skin. When assessing skin turgor, explain the procedure to the patient and gently pinch their skin between the thumb and forefinger, observing how quickly it returns to its original position. Failure to spring back may indicate dehydration.

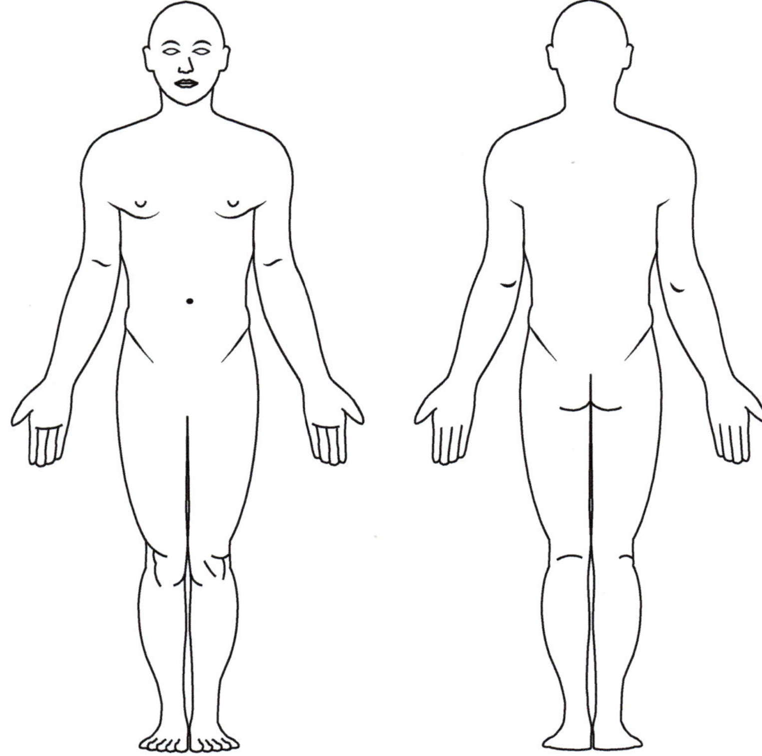

FIGURE 2.3 Body map

Upon completion of the examination, assist the patient in changing back into their clothes, wash hands, report findings and document them in accordance with local policies and procedures. Body mapping can aid in documenting findings, with computerised digital imaging systems and total body mapping photography providing objective monitoring of lesions. Alternatively, a basic line-drawn body map can be used for documentation purposes (see Figure 2.3).

Findings that are based on the patient history and the physical examination can assist in making a diagnosis and then for the formulation of an individual plan of care for the patient. The findings can also assist in the ordering of further tests and investigations if a definitive diagnosis needs confirmation.

PSYCHODERMATOLOGY

Psychodermatology focuses on the interaction between psychological factors and skin disorders. It explores the relationship between mental health and skin conditions, recognising the impact they can have on each other. Psychodermatology encompasses various aspects, including understanding how psychological stressors can exacerbate skin conditions, the psychological effects of living with a skin disorder and the role of psychological interventions in managing skin conditions. It involves interdisciplinary collaboration between dermatologists, psychologists, psychiatrists and other healthcare professionals to provide comprehensive care for patients with both skin and psychological concerns.

As the skin is the largest organ in the body and the one most commonly looked at by healthcare professionals and other people, the impact of a skin disorder on a patient's life and their family can be significant. Emotional trauma can occur from the development of a number of skin conditions, including psoriasis, atopic eczema, discoid eczema, alopecia areata and urticaria. The impact of emotional trauma can lead to stress, low self-esteem, social isolation, depression and in some cases suicide. Self-image and quality of life can be severely affected by a skin disorder as the scarring can be both physical and psychological, such as that witnessed in acne vulgaris. It must also be remembered that psychological illnesses, for example, depression, anxiety and stress, have the potential to trigger or exacerbate a skin disorder. Mukwende et al. (2020) notes that within psychodermatology, four groupings have been identified:

1. Psychophysiological: emotional stress triggering inflammatory responses in the skin.

2. Primary psychiatric: self-induced injury of the skin (iatrogenic).

3. Secondary psychiatric: emotional effects arising from a pre-existing skin condition, such as anxiety, frustration and depression.

4. Cutaneous sensory disorders: individuals with no evident skin or medical conditions may experience unpleasant skin sensations such as itching, soreness and pain, alongside adverse sensory symptoms such as numbness and hypoesthesia.

Diagnosing a skin disorder primarily involves a thorough inspection of the skin.

The physical examination and data recording must be undertaken in a systematic manner with attention to description and detail regarding skin findings, including nails and hair. Following the collection of primary and secondary data, a preliminary diagnosis can often be reached. However, to confirm a definitive diagnosis, further tests and investigations may be necessary.

CONCLUSION

Understanding the functions of the skin and its various structures can enable those who offer care and support in the delivery of evidence-based care. Proficiency in recognising the various structures of the skin and their functions, along with refined assessment techniques can assist in effectively addressing patient needs and intervening when issues arise. A systematic approach to skin history and physical examination is emphasised in caring for individuals with skin disorders.

The skin is an extraordinary organ. It serves as a window to various diseases and injuries, manifesting symptoms such as rashes, jaundice or cyanosis. As the largest organ in terms of weight and surface area, it also reflects emotional states, evidenced by phenomena such as blushing, sweating and trembling. Its accessibility makes it prone to injury, including infections and trauma.

GLOSSARY OF TERMS

Alopecia: Partial or complete hair loss.

Bulla: A large blister or vesicle filled with fluid.

Cyanosis: Bluish discolouration of the skin due to lack of oxygen.

Dermatitis: Inflammation of the skin.

Eczema: A chronic skin condition characterised by red, itchy and inflamed skin.

Exudate: Fluid, such as pus or serum, that oozes from a wound or inflamed skin.

Jaundice: Yellow discolouration of the skin and eyes due to liver dysfunction.

Lesion: Abnormality or damage in the skin, such as a rash, sore or ulcer.

Macule: Flat, discoloured spot on the skin.

Nodule: Solid, raised lesion or lump in the skin.

Pallor: Unnatural paleness of the skin.

Papule: Small, raised bump on the skin.

Petechiae: Tiny, red or purple spots on the skin caused by bleeding under the skin.

Pruritus: Itching sensation of the skin.

Purpura: Purple or red discolouration of the skin caused by bleeding under the skin.

Pustule: Small, pus-filled blister or bump on the skin.

Rash: Change in the colour or texture of the skin due to inflammation or infection.

Scar: Mark left on the skin after a wound has healed.

Vesicle: Small blister filled with clear fluid.

MULTIPLE CHOICE QUESTIONS

1. Which of the following terms refers to a chronic skin condition characterised by red, itchy and inflamed skin?
   a) Psoriasis
   b) Eczema
   c) Acne
   d) Dermatitis

2. What is the primary cause of cyanosis?
   a) Excessive sweating
   b) Lack of oxygen in the blood
   c) Liver dysfunction
   d) High blood pressure

3. Petechiae are tiny, red or purple spots on the skin caused by:
   a) Allergic reactions
   b) Excessive sun exposure
   c) Bleeding under the skin
   d) Bacterial infections

4. What is the medical term for itching sensation of the skin?
   a) Pruritus
   b) Pallor
   c) Purpura
   d) Pustule

5. Which skin condition is characterised by unnatural paleness of the skin?
   a) Jaundice
   b) Dermatitis
   c) Pallor
   d) Eczema

6. Which of the following terms refers to a flat, discoloured spot on the skin?
   a) Macule
   b) Nodule
   c) Vesicle
   d) Bulla

7. Exudate refers to:
   a) Fluid, such as pus or serum, that oozes from a wound or inflamed skin
   b) Small, pus-filled blister or bump on the skin
   c) Solid, raised lesion or lump in the skin
   d) Red or purple spots on the skin caused by bleeding under the skin

8. What term is used for excessive hair growth, particularly in females, in areas where males usually have hair?
   a) Alopecia
   b) Hirsutism
   c) Hypoesthesia
   d) Petechiae

9. What is the primary cause of jaundice?
   a) Lack of oxygen in the blood
   b) Liver dysfunction
   c) Allergic reactions
   d) Excessive sweating

10. What is the term for a chronic inflammatory skin condition characterised by red, itchy and scaly patches?
    a) Psoriasis
    b) Eczema
    c) Dermatitis
    d) Acne

REFERENCES

Bickley, L.S., Szilagyi, P.G. and Hoffman, R.M. (eds) (2024). *Bates' Guide to Physical Examination and History Taking*, 13e. Philadelphia: Wolters Kluwer.

McPhillips, H., Wood, A.F., Harper-MacDonald, B. et al. (2021). Conducting a consultation and clinical assessment of the skin for advanced clinical practitioners. *British Journal of Nursing* 30 (21): 1232–1236.

Mukwende, M., Tamony, P. and Turner, M. (2020). *Mind the Gap: A Handbook of Clinical Signs in Black and Brown Skin*. University of London, London: St George's.

Peters, J. (2019). Nursing patients with skin disorders (Chapter 13). In: *Alexander's Nursing Practice*, 6e. (ed. I. Peate). London: Elsevier.

Stephens, M. (2022). The principles of skin integrity (Chapter 18). In: *Nursing Practice*, 3e. (eds. I. Peate and A. Mitchell). Oxford: Wiley.

Rhoads, J. and Wiggins Petersen, S. (2021). *Advanced Health Assessment and Diagnostic Reasoning*, 4e. Burlington: Jones and Bartlett.

Tidman, M.J. (2018). The skin, hair and nails (Chapter 14). In: *Macleod's Clinical Examination*, 14e. (eds. J.A. Innes, A.R. Dover and K. Fairhurst). Edinburgh: Elsevier.

World Union of Wound Healing Societies (2019). Wound exudate effective assessment and management. https://www.wuwhs.org/wp-content/uploads/2020/09/exudate.pdf (accessed May 2024).

Chronic skin conditions can impact individuals of all ages and persist throughout their lives. Many skin disorders, such as psoriasis, eczema, acne, vitiligo, leg ulcers and damage from chronic sun exposure, leading to multiple skin cancers are chronic conditions. Some chronic skin conditions have lasting physical and psychological effects. Psoriasis, for instance, can result in enduring disabilities and challenges in personal relationships and employment prospects. Psoriasis is not a contagious condition.

Skin disorders rank among the top reasons for seeking medical advice in primary care. They significantly contribute to the burden of chronic conditions. There is a widespread prevalence of chronic skin disorders such as psoriasis, eczema, acne, vitiligo and skin conditions that are caused by occupational exposure. Beyond these dermatological issues, many other chronic health conditions require substantial dermatological care. This could be either because the illness is affecting the person's skin directly or it may be due to the medications that are used to treat the condition and their associated side effects. Specific dermatological conditions, particularly psoriasis, are associated with significant additional health problems that are known as comorbidities. In the case of psoriasis, these comorbidities include conditions such as metabolic syndrome (a cluster of conditions that increase the risk of heart disease, stroke and type 2 diabetes), arthritis and depression. In essence, it highlights the interconnectedness of dermatological health with overall health and well-being.

Griffiths et al. (2021) describe psoriasis as a common condition, a chronic papulosquamous skin disease that affects people globally. The condition can present at any age, and it leads to a considerable burden for individuals and society.

TYPES OF PSORIASIS

Psoriasis can manifest in several different forms, each with its own characteristics and symptoms (Castro 2019).

PLAQUE PSORIASIS

This is the most common form of psoriasis. It is characterised by raised, red patches of skin covered with silvery-white scales, known as plaques. These plaques can appear anywhere on the body, but they are most commonly found on the elbows, knees, scalp and lower back.

GUTTATE PSORIASIS

Guttate psoriasis often starts in childhood or young adulthood and is characterised by small, red, scaly spots that appear on the skin, typically on the trunk, limbs and scalp. It is often triggered by bacterial infections, such as Group A Streptococcus bacteria.

INVERSE PSORIASIS

Inverse psoriasis affects skin folds, such as those in the armpits, groin, under the breasts and around the genitals. It appears as smooth, red patches of inflamed skin that may be more sensitive and prone to irritation due to friction and sweating.

PUSTULAR PSORIASIS

This type of psoriasis is characterised by raised, pus-filled bumps (pustules) that are surrounded by red skin. The skin around the pustules is usually red and tender. Pustular psoriasis can be localised to certain areas of the body or generalised where it can cover large areas.

ERYTHRODERMIC PSORIASIS

Erythrodermic psoriasis is a severe and rare form of psoriasis that can affect the entire body. It causes a widespread redness, severe itching and shedding of scales in sheets, which resembles a severe sunburn. Erythrodermic psoriasis can be life-threatening and requires immediate medical attention (see Figure 3.1).

NAIL PSORIASIS

Psoriasis can also affect the nails, which causes changes such as pitting, discolouration, thickening and separation from the nail bed. Nail psoriasis can be challenging to treat and may cause discomfort and difficulty in performing everyday tasks (see Figure 3.2).

SCALP PSORIASIS

This can range from mild to severe and its symptoms can vary from person to person. While it may not always be the most visible form of psoriasis, it can still cause discomfort and affect the

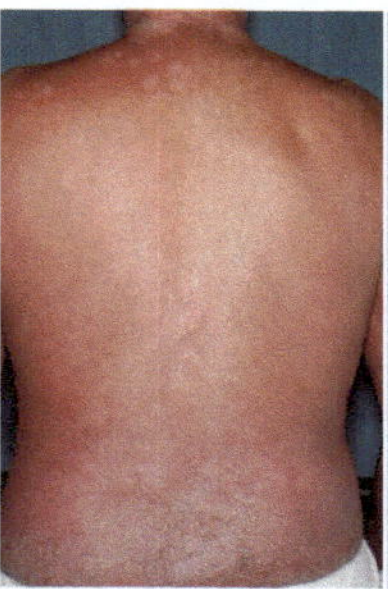

FIGURE 3.1   Erythrodermic psoriasis. *Source:* Chowdhury et al. (2021). With permission from John Wiley & Sons.

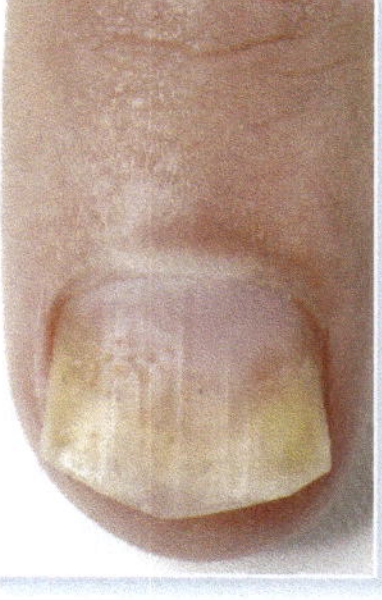

FIGURE 3.2   Nail psoriasis with yellow separation and pitting of the nail. *Source:* Chowdhury et al. (2021). With permission from John Wiley & Sons.

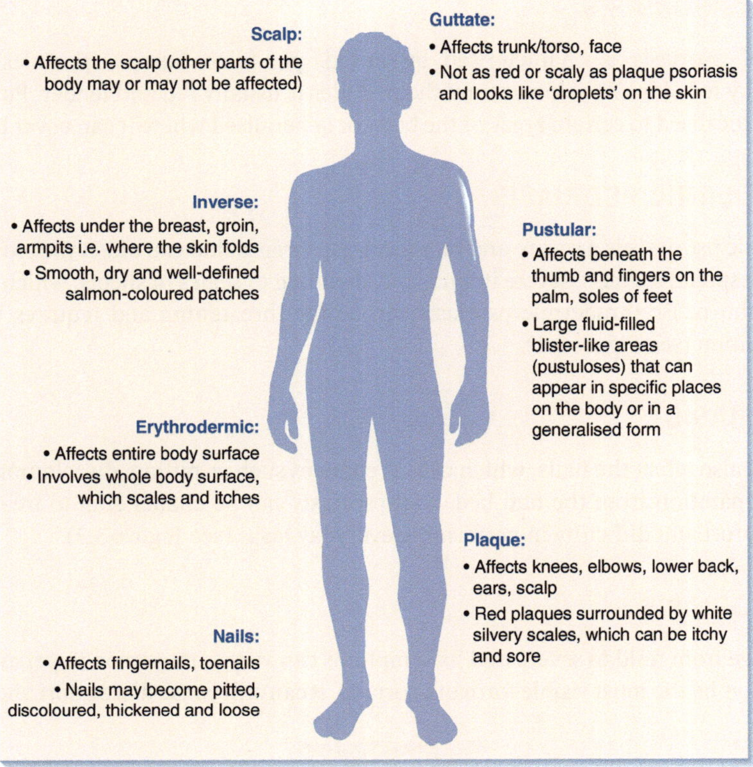

FIGURE 3.3 Types of psoriasis

quality of life due to the symptoms that may include itching, scaling and sometimes temporary hair loss.

These are just some of the forms of psoriasis and individuals may experience a combination of these types or different forms over time, see Figure 3.3. Collaborating closely with healthcare professionals is crucial for individuals with psoriasis to effectively manage their condition and reduce its impact on their quality of life. Additionally, those who provide care and support must be responsive to the needs of people with psoriasis. Understanding the different types of psoriasis is important as it helps healthcare professionals accurately diagnose the condition. Treatment choices can then be tailored to meet individual needs, monitor for potential complications, offer information and advice to patients about their condition and treatment options and contribute to ongoing research efforts aimed at improving therapies and outcomes.

PATHOPHYSIOLOGICAL CHANGES ASSOCIATED WITH PSORIASIS

Psoriasis is a complex autoimmune disorder that is characterised by dysregulation of the immune system, which leads to chronic inflammation and abnormal skin cell growth. The pathophysiological changes associated with psoriasis involve interactions between immune cells, genetic factors, environmental triggers and skin cells.

In psoriasis, the immune system becomes excessively active, with specific involvement of T cells, dendritic cells and certain cytokines (such as tumour necrosis factor-alpha, interleukin-17 and interleukin-23). These are immune cells and they become overly sensitive. This results in persistent inflammation and the release of substances that promote inflammation.

Genetic factors play a significant role in the development of psoriasis. There are several genes associated with immune function, skin barrier integrity and inflammation that have been implicated in psoriasis susceptibility. However, it is important to note that not everyone with these genetic predispositions will develop psoriasis, indicating that environmental factors also play a role. There are various environmental factors that can trigger or exacerbate psoriasis flare-ups in genetically susceptible individuals.

One of the hallmarks of psoriasis is the excessive proliferation of keratinocytes (skin cells) in the epidermis. Normally, skin cells will go through a cycle of growth and shedding over the course of about a month. In psoriasis, this process is accelerated, with the skin cells turning over every few days instead. This rapid turnover leads to the formation of thickened patches of skin (plaques) characteristic of psoriasis.

Psoriasis is also associated with increased blood vessel formation (angiogenesis) and the development of new blood vessels (neovascularisation) in the skin. This enhanced vascularisation contributes to the redness and inflammation that is observed in psoriatic plaques.

The inflammation that is observed in psoriasis is driven by a complex interaction between different types of immune cells and signalling molecules called cytokines. Activated T cells travel to the skin and release cytokines; these trigger inflammation and attract more immune cells to the affected area. This ongoing cycle of inflammation leads to tissue damage, further immune system activation and rapid proliferation of skin cells, contributing to the characteristic symptoms of psoriasis.

Psoriasis is a multifactorial disorder that involves genetic predisposition, immune dysregulation, environmental triggers and abnormal skin cell proliferation and inflammation. Understanding these pathophysiological changes is important for developing targeted therapies that are aimed at controlling inflammation, restoring skin barrier function and improving the quality of life for individuals with psoriasis.

While symptoms often remain mild, there are some individuals who may experience intense itching. This condition may have significant cosmetic implications. Additionally, psoriatic arthritis, a progressive type of inflammatory arthritis (Hagler et al. 2023) (see Figure 3.4) may develop in some people. Diagnosis usually relies on the appearance and distribution of the skin lesions. There are a range of treatment options available. Primary Care Dermatology Society (2023) notes that psoriasis cannot be cured and achieving complete clearance may not always be feasible. However, numerous effective treatments that are available to manage psoriasis. It is rare for psoriasis to spontaneously clear.

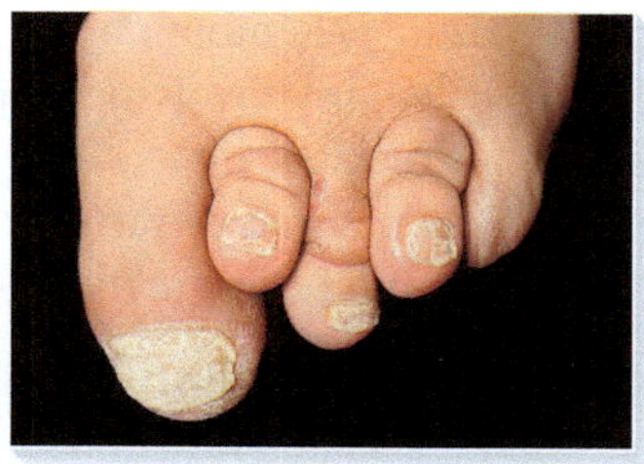

FIGURE 3.4 Psoriatic arthritis

EPIDEMIOLOGY

Although psoriasis is a frequently occurring skin condition, its true extent may be underestimated since individuals with mild symptoms might not seek medical advice, which potentially skews prevalence and incidence data.

The prevalence of psoriasis is estimated to be around 1.3–2.2% in the UK. Psoriasis can occur at any age, although it is uncommon in children (0.71%) and most cases occur before 35 years. Men and women are equally affected. Psoriasis is associated with joint disease in a significant proportion of patients (reported in one study at 13.8%). Plaque psoriasis is by far the most common form of the condition (about 90% of people with psoriasis). Distinctive nail changes occur in around 50% of all those affected and are more common in people with psoriatic arthritis (National Institute for Health and Care Excellence [NICE] 2017). While psoriasis can occur in people of any ethnic background, there are variations in prevalence among different ethnic groups (Johnson and Armstrong 2013). There is a higher likelihood among individuals of White ethnicity compared to other racial groups.

There are regional variances in psoriasis prevalence within the UK. Urban areas, industrialised regions and areas with higher pollution levels may exhibit higher rates of psoriasis. This is perhaps due to environmental triggers and lifestyle factors.

Epidemiological and demographic data play a pivotal role in understanding the backdrop to psoriasis in the UK and are essential for guiding various public health initiatives and healthcare interventions aimed at improving outcomes for affected individuals. The data provide valuable insights and have the potential to contribute to efforts in raising awareness, improving access to care and developing effective treatment strategies, and to mitigate the impact of psoriasis on individuals, families and communities.

RISK FACTORS

Psoriasis is a multifaceted condition that is influenced by a combination of genetic predisposition, environmental triggers and immune system dysregulation (Peters 2019). Recognising the various risk factors that are linked to psoriasis can aid in identifying individuals who may be at higher risk of developing the disorder.

Family history plays a significant role in psoriasis risk. The National Psoriasis Foundation (2022) reports that individuals with a parent affected by psoriasis face a 28% likelihood of developing the condition themselves. Should both parents have psoriasis, the risk escalates to 65%. Multiple genes have been implicated in psoriasis susceptibility, with variations in certain genes affecting immune function and skin cell turnover.

Kamiya et al. (2019) discuss a range of risk factors associated with the development of psoriasis. Psoriasis is considered an autoimmune disorder, where the immune system mistakenly attacks healthy skin cells. This leads to inflammation and the rapid growth of skin cells. Dysregulation of immune pathways, particularly involving T cells and cytokines, contributes to the development and progression of psoriasis.

There are various environmental factors that can trigger or exacerbate psoriasis symptoms in susceptible individuals. These common triggers include:

- Bacterial or viral infections, such as streptococcal throat infections, can trigger psoriasis flare-ups. Streptococcal infection is strongly associated with guttate psoriasis, especially with upper respiratory tract infection and may also be a trigger for or exacerbate chronic plaque psoriasis. Infection can also precipitate generalised pustular psoriasis or erythrodermic psoriasis.

- Physical trauma to the skin, such as cuts, scratches, piercings, tattoos and burns, can trigger psoriasis lesions in susceptible individuals. This is known as the Koebner phenomenon.

- Psychological stress and emotional upheaval can exacerbate psoriasis symptoms or trigger flare-ups in some individuals.

- Certain medications, such as lithium, antimalarial drugs, beta-blockers and non-steroidal anti-inflammatory drugs, angiotensin-converting enzyme inhibitors, and antibiotics, such as tetracycline and penicillin, can worsen psoriasis symptoms or induce psoriasis-like skin lesions in predisposed individuals. Sudden oral or potent topical corticosteroid withdrawal can lead to a severe rebound phenomenon and can evolve into generalised pustular psoriasis or erythrodermic psoriasis.

- Tobacco smoking and excessive alcohol consumption have been associated with an increased risk of developing psoriasis and exacerbating existing symptoms.

- Ultraviolet (UV) light exposure and sunlight are usually beneficial, but they may exacerbate psoriasis in some people and can precipitate generalised pustular psoriasis.

There is growing evidence linking obesity, insulin resistance and metabolic syndrome with an increased risk of psoriasis. Obesity is associated with chronic low-grade inflammation, which may exacerbate immune dysregulation and contribute to psoriasis development or severity.

Hormonal changes, such as those occurring during puberty, pregnancy or menopause, can influence psoriasis symptoms. Some women experience improvement in psoriasis during pregnancy, while others may notice worsening symptoms postpartum or during menopause.

Recognising these risk factors can help improve the assessment of an individual's likelihood of developing psoriasis and to tailor preventive measures, lifestyle modifications and treatment approaches accordingly. Additionally, understanding these factors contributes to ongoing research efforts aimed at elucidating the underlying mechanisms of psoriasis and developing targeted therapies for improved management of the condition.

CLINICAL PRESENTATION

The clinical presentation of psoriasis can vary widely among affected individuals, but certain hallmark features are typically observed. The disease most commonly manifests on the skin of the elbows, knees, scalp, lumbosacral areas, intergluteal clefts and genitalia (see Figure 3.5). Plaques typically appear in the same areas on both sides of the body. For example, if one knee or elbow is covered, the other is also affected (National Psoriasis Foundation 2024).

Chowdhury, Katugampola, and Finlay (2019) discuss clinical presentations. Psoriasis presents with numerous patches of reddened, slightly elevated and scaly skin known as 'plaques'. These plaques usually exhibit well-defined borders and often occur symmetrically across the body. Figure 3.6 demonstrates the typical plaques associated with psoriasis and Figure 3.7 demonstrates guttate psoriasis. When irritated, the plaques tend to bleed more readily than unaffected skin. Commonly affected areas include the knees, elbows and scalp, although any part of the body can be involved. These lesions persist for extended periods and may slowly expand and merge, often causing itching. Patients are mainly troubled by the visible appearance, the presence of scales and the profound disruption that the condition can impose on their daily lives. See Box 3.1, psoriasis morphology refers to the physical characteristics and appearance of psoriasis lesions or plaques. It encompasses various aspects such as the colour, texture, distribution and arrangement of the skin lesions associated with psoriasis.

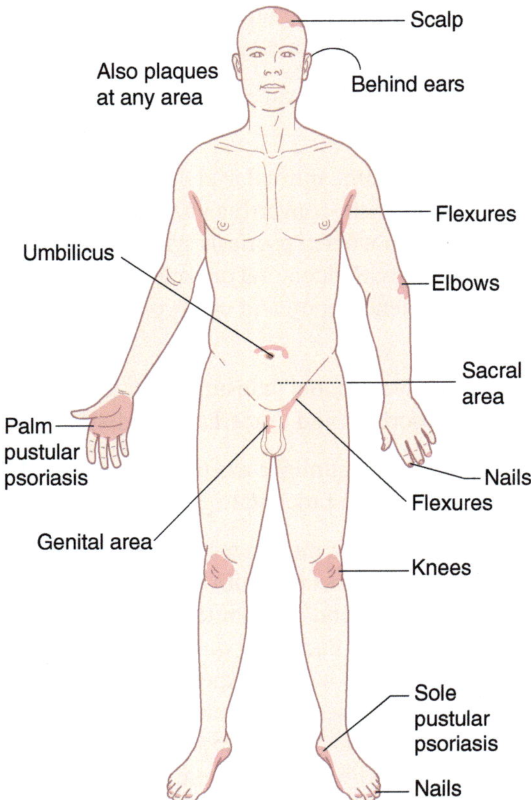

FIGURE 3.5 Common locations of psoriasis

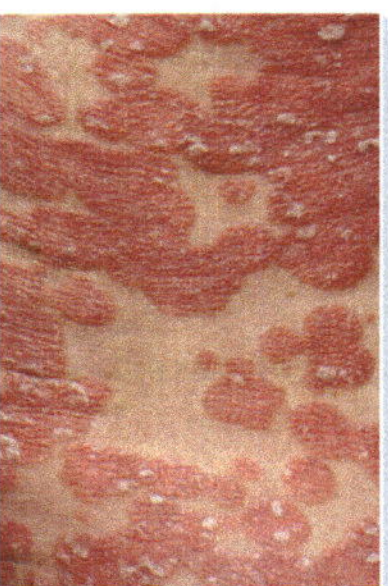

FIGURE 3.6 Typical plaques of psoriasis. *Source:* Chowdhury et al. (2021). With permission from John Wiley & Sons.

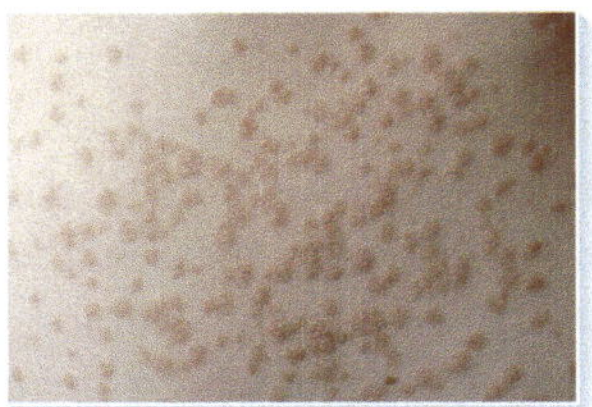

FIGURE 3.7 Guttate psoriasis: multiple small lesions. *Source:* Chowdhury et al. (2021). With permission from John Wiley & Sons.

BOX 3.1	PSORIASIS MORPHOLOGY

- Most cases of chronic plaque psoriasis are described as large plaque psoriasis or small plaque psoriasis.

- Plaques are ruby-red and well-defined with a silvery surface scale on lighter skin tones. On darker skin, they may appear salmon-coloured, dark brown, purple or violet with greyish scales. People with darker skin might also have more scaling, more affected skin areas and skin lesions misdiagnosed as hyperpigmentation (patches of darker skin).

- The plaques can join together to involve very extensive areas of the skin, particularly when on the trunk and limbs.

- Auspitz sign refers to a clinical phenomenon that is observed in psoriasis, where scraping or picking off adherent psoriatic scales leads to pinpoint bleeding. The bleeding results from the rupture of capillaries that undulate vertically within the thickened skin characteristic of psoriasis lesions. The presence of the Auspitz sign is considered a diagnostic feature of psoriasis and is indicative of the intense vascularity and abnormal skin architecture that is associated with the condition.

- Auspitz sign: when adherent psoriatic scales are scraped or picked off pinpoint bleeding, these are known as the Auspitz sign. They may occur from capillaries, which undulate vertically throughout the thickened psoriatic skin.

- Lesions on the lower legs may be less typical.

Source: Primary Care Dermatology Society (2023); National Psoriasis Foundation Skin of Color Resource Center (psoriasis.org).

In areas such as the groin, axillae or other skin folds where there is psoriasis, the scales tend to detach easily due to moisture, which results in a shiny red appearance. Scalp psoriasis may be felt more than is visible. Upon parting the hair, however, greyish matted scales are seen as opposed to the usual appearance of the scalp skin. Scalp psoriasis usually demonstrates well-defined borders, often with areas unaffected, distinguishing it from dandruff, which affects the entire scalp uniformly.

It is important to be aware of the signs and symptoms of psoriatic arthritis in people with psoriasis, such as joint pain, swelling, stiffness and reduced range of movement. Early detection and management of psoriatic arthritis is essential for preventing joint damage and preserving joint function.

CLINICAL INVESTIGATIONS AND DIAGNOSIS

Skin irritation, a rash or flaky, dry skin that lasts longer than a few weeks, would indicate that the patient should consult a healthcare professional. To make a diagnosis of psoriasis, a combination of clinical evaluation and in some cases, supportive laboratory or imaging investigations are required. A medical history is taken and an examination of the skin, nails and scalp is undertaken and if appropriate the joints (Psoriasis Association 2023). Other investigations and tests may also be required to distinguish psoriasis from other skin diseases.

PSORIASIS AREA AND SEVERITY INDEX

Psoriasis severity is assessed at various stages: at initial diagnosis, prior to specialist referral, during specialist consultations and to gauge treatment effectiveness. There are a number of scoring systems that can be used to evaluate psoriasis severity. This includes skin and joint involvement, impact on mood and daily activities and potential cardiovascular risk. One assessment tool is the Psoriasis Area and Severity Index (PASI) score (Feldman and Kruege 2005). PASI is a widely used tool in dermatology. It aims to assess the severity of psoriasis and monitor treatment response over time. It provides a standardised method for quantifying the extent and severity of psoriasis lesions based on objective criteria. The PASI evaluates four key parameters:

1. Erythema (redness): The degree of redness or inflammation present in psoriasis lesions is assessed on a scale from 0 to 4, with 0 indicating no redness and 4 indicating severe redness.

2. Induration (thickness): The thickness or elevation of psoriasis plaques is evaluated on a scale from 0 to 4, with 0 indicating no thickening and 4 indicating severe thickening.

3. Desquamation (scaling): The amount of scaling or flaking of the skin within psoriasis lesions is graded on a scale from 0 to 4, with 0 indicating no scaling and 4 indicating severe scaling.

4. Percentage of body surface area (BSA) affected: The extent of psoriasis involvement is estimated based on the percentage of BSA affected by psoriasis lesions. The body is divided into specific regions and the percentage involvement of each region is assessed and recorded.

The PASI score is calculated using a formula that incorporates the individual scores for erythema, induration and desquamation in each region of the body, along with the percentage of BSA involvement. The total PASI score ranges from 0 to 72, with higher scores indicating greater disease severity.

HISTORY TAKING

Skin disease's visibility might lead to the assumption that a patient's history is unnecessary. However, obtaining an accurate patient history is fundamental to quality care. Neglecting a thorough history could result in overlooking crucial information. Knowing the history of the current condition and treatment response guides care effectively. Simply examining the skin does not reveal the extent of its impact on the patient's life. Awareness of the medications the patient is taking is important as some may exacerbate or contraindicate use. Family history is important for genetic or infectious considerations. Understanding the influence of the patient's work on the condition and vice versa is vital for holistic care. Identifying associated conditions aids in comprehensive patient evaluation. Assessing the psychological impact, including concerns about prescribed medication or planned procedures, demonstrates supportive care.

A structured history involves the following steps:

Introductions

- Initiate introductions to establish rapport.

Current Complaint

- Use general open-ended questions to explore the patient's concern(s).
- Determine onset, course and main symptoms of the condition.
- Identify affected areas and factors that may exacerbate or alleviate symptoms.

Past Medical History

- Inquire about prior skin conditions, including common ones such as eczema, psoriasis and acne.

- Explore systemic diseases with skin manifestations, such as diabetes, tuberculosis, immunosuppression or HIV.

Drugs and Allergies

- Document current and past use of both topical and systemic medications.

- Investigate previous treatments for skin conditions and their efficacy.

- Assess for potential contact allergies or systemic drug allergies.

- Note any history of immediate allergies, such as latex.

Social History

- Evaluate the impact of the skin disease on the patient's daily life and occupation.

- Consider the influence of occupation on the skin condition.

- Inquire about alcohol consumption and smoking habits, which may affect certain skin conditions.

- Explore the history of high sun exposure or sunbed use, which could impact the skin.

Family History

- Explore family history of eczema, asthma, hay fever, psoriasis, genetic diseases or skin cancer.

- Note any genetic predispositions or familial patterns related to the patient's skin condition.

Table 3.1 provides a summary of history taking.

Obtaining a comprehensive medical history encompassing the components highlighted in Table 3.1 can help to effectively diagnose psoriasis, differentiate it from other skin conditions, assess disease severity and develop personalised treatment plans that are tailored to the individual patient's needs. Understanding the psychosocial impact and associated comorbidities of psoriasis is integral to providing holistic patient-centred care.

Table 3.1 History taking

Component	Content	Discussion
Onset and duration of symptoms	Inquire about when the skin symptoms first appeared and how they have progressed over time.	Understanding the timeline of symptom onset helps differentiate psoriasis from other skin conditions and provides insights into disease progression.
Previous diagnoses and treatments	Explore any previous diagnoses or treatments for psoriasis or other skin conditions.	This includes inquiring about prior topical or systemic medications, phototherapy or other therapies used to manage skin symptoms.

(Continued)

Table 3.1 (*Continued*)

Component	Content	Discussion
Family history of psoriasis	Investigating the family history of psoriasis is essential, as genetics play a significant role in predisposing individuals to the condition.	A positive family history increases the likelihood of developing psoriasis and may influence disease severity and treatment response.
Triggers and exacerbating factors	Explore potential triggers or exacerbating factors that may precipitate or worsen psoriasis symptoms. These may include stress, infections, certain medications or environmental exposures.	Identifying and addressing these triggers can help manage and prevent psoriasis flare-ups.
Psychosocial impact	Assessing the psychosocial impact of psoriasis is essential for understanding its holistic impact on the patient's quality of life.	Healthcare providers inquire about the emotional and social implications of living with psoriasis, including feelings of embarrassment, self-consciousness or depression.
Associated conditions	Psoriasis is associated with several comorbidities, including psoriatic arthritis, cardiovascular disease, metabolic syndrome and autoimmune disorders.	Inquiring about any associated conditions or symptoms may influence treatment decisions and overall management.
Medication history	In addition to exploring previous treatments for psoriasis, an assessment of the patient's current and past medication history is made.	Certain medications, such as beta-blockers, lithium or antimalarials, may exacerbate psoriasis or trigger flare-ups. Determine over-the-counter use of medications.

Source: Adapted from Chowdhury, Katugampola, and Finlay (2019).

USE OF PHOTOGRAPHY

Photography can play an important role in the assessment of skin, serving various purposes such as documenting and monitoring skin conditions, educating patients and aiding in diagnosis (Mattessich and Grant-Kels 2020). It is crucial, however, to conduct clinical photography in a manner that respects patient privacy and ensures that their consent has been obtained. Patients should be informed about the purpose of the photographs and how they will be used with their consent obtained beforehand. Signed patient permission is required and the copy is kept in their notes. Separate permissions are needed for teaching, publication or use on the internet. A personal camera or a mobile phone camera should not be used; the use of a dedicated clinical camera is advocated. Unless essential, do not take photographs where the patient can be recognised.

Clinical photography enables the visual documentation of a patient's skin condition at a specific moment, facilitating the tracking of condition progression or treatment effectiveness over time. High-quality photographs can assist in diagnosing skin conditions by providing a visual record that can be referenced later or shared with other healthcare professionals for additional insights or opinions. Photographs help patients understand their skin conditions more effectively, allowing them to visualise what is being described. This visual aid often leads to improved treatment compliance and better patient understanding.

PHYSICAL EXAMINATION

A physical examination is essential in making a diagnosis of psoriasis because it helps to directly observe and assess the characteristic symptoms and signs of the condition. Classifying the type of psoriasis will guide management, where possible, assess skin lesions over the whole body (NICE 2017). Psoriasis typically presents with distinct features on the skin, such as red, inflamed patches covered with silvery scales. These symptoms often appear in specific areas of the body, such as the elbows, knees, scalp and lower back, but they can also affect other parts of the body.

Prior to the examination, the rationale for it and how it will proceed must be explained to the patient. The patient should be positioned in such a way that the skin can be examined, ensuring the patient is comfortable only to expose the relevant areas. Ensure privacy, offer a chaperone and document the outcome of this; the willingness of the patient to be examined is gained through informed consent and all policies and procedures related to infection, prevention and control must be adhered to. Asses vital signs, weight and height; it is essential to have a good light source, a ruler, a magnifying glass and a dermatoscope available (Figure 3.8).

Adopting a systematic approach to physical examination is essential for ensuring thorough, accurate and efficient patient assessment, leading to better outcomes and quality of care. Chowdhury, Katugampola, and Finlay (2019) suggest an initial head-to-toe approach (see Figure 3.9).

The examination can reveal a disease process that is limited exclusively to the skin or indicate a broader systemic condition. Skin lesions come in diverse forms and a thorough examination aids in discerning whether the findings are localised to the skin or indicative of

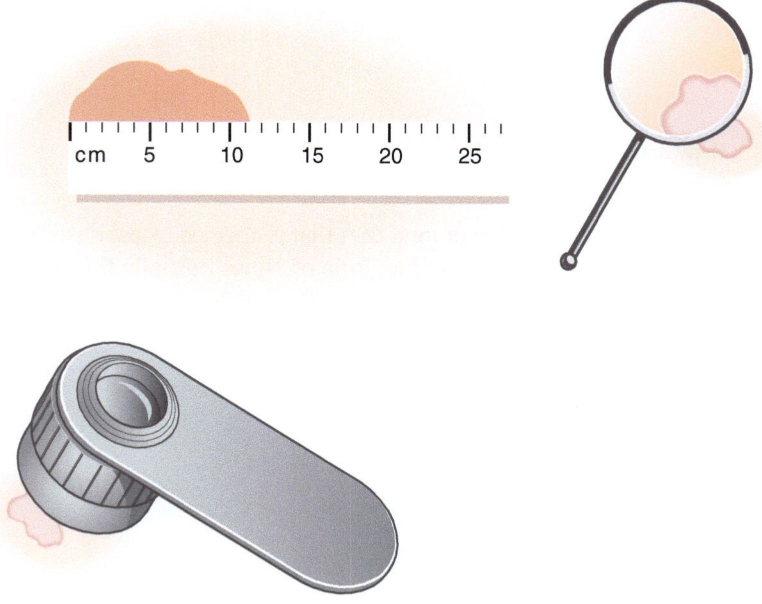

FIGURE 3.8   A ruler, a magnifying glass and a dermatoscope

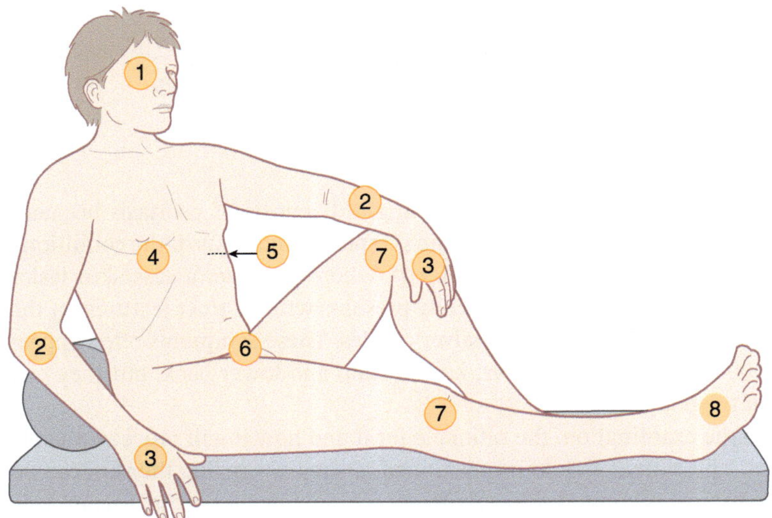

FIGURE 3.9 A head-to-toe approach

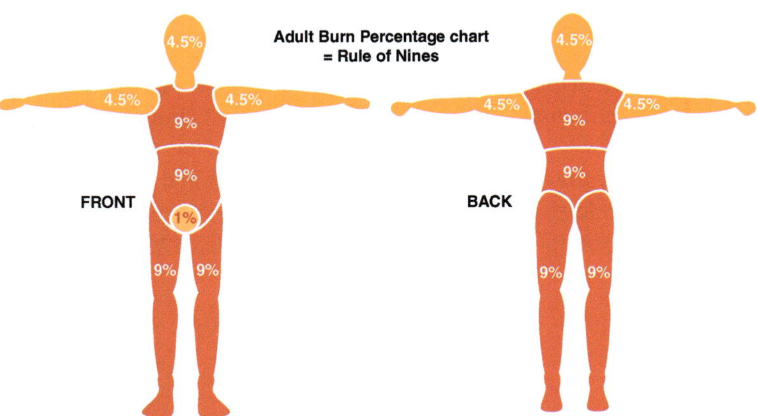

FIGURE 3.10 Body map

systemic involvement. The proportion of total BSA that is affected by psoriasis is assessed and documented. This can be estimated using the 'Rule of Nines' (usually this is used for burns assessment).

Estimates of BSA:

Arm: 9%

Head: 9%

Neck: 1%

Leg: 18%

Anterior trunk: 18%

Posterior trunk: 18%

A body map should be used to document findings (see Figure 3.10).

Table 3.2   The physical examination

Component	Discussion
Detailed inspection of skin lesions	During the physical examination, healthcare providers conduct a thorough evaluation of the skin, paying close attention to any visible lesions. Psoriasis lesions typically manifest as well-defined, raised plaques with a characteristic red colour and silvery-white scales. These plaques may vary in size, shape and distribution, commonly appearing on extensor surfaces such as the elbows and knees. However, they can also affect other areas of the body, including the scalp, lower back, palms, soles of the feet and nails.
Assessment of lesion distribution and extent	A careful assessment is made of the distribution and extent of psoriasis lesions across the body. The presence of localised lesions, widespread involvement or specific patterns of distribution, such as symmetric involvement of bilateral joints, are noted. Lesions may occur singly or in clusters and their distribution can vary depending on the subtype of psoriasis and individual patient characteristics.
Evaluation of lesion severity	The severity of psoriasis lesions is evaluated based on several factors, including the size, thickness, erythema and scaling of the plaques. Standardised assessment tools such as the PASI are used to quantify the severity of psoriasis lesions objectively. These tools help monitor disease progression over time, assess treatment response and guide therapeutic decisions.
Assessment of associated symptoms	In addition to visual inspection, inquire about any associated symptoms experienced by the patient, such as itching, pain or bleeding from the lesions. Itching, in particular, is a common symptom of psoriasis and can significantly impact the patient's quality of life. Pain or discomfort may occur, especially in areas where lesions are located over joints or in areas prone to friction or irritation.
Examination of psoriatic nail changes	Psoriasis can affect the nails, causing characteristic changes such as pitting, ridges, discolouration, thickening, crumbling or separation from the nail bed. The nails are carefully examined for signs of psoriatic nail involvement, as these changes can be indicative of the severity of the underlying skin disease and may require specific management strategies.
Scalp examination	For patients with suspected scalp psoriasis, the hair is parted and the scalp is examined for signs of redness, scaling, plaques or other abnormalities. Scalp psoriasis can be challenging to diagnose visually, especially in patients with thick hair or mild disease activity. In such cases, a thorough examination of the scalp and close inspection of any scaling or erythema beneath the hairline are essential for accurate diagnosis and appropriate management.

Source: Adapted from NICE (2017); Primary Care Dermatology Society (2023).

Table 3.2 provides a summary of the components related to physical examination. The details of the physical examination must be responsive to the patient's individual needs.

INVESTIGATIONS

In some cases, a skin biopsy may be performed to confirm the diagnosis, especially if the presentation is atypical or other skin conditions need to be ruled out (Peters 2019). During a biopsy, a small sample of skin tissue is taken from a psoriasis lesion and this is examined under a microscope by a pathologist.

Depending on the clinical presentation and suspected complications, additional tests may be ordered. These may include blood tests to assess for markers of inflammation (e.g. C-reactive protein, erythrocyte sedimentation rate), screening for associated conditions (such as psoriatic arthritis, metabolic syndrome) or ruling out infections.

Performing a comprehensive physical examination can help to effectively identify characteristic features of psoriasis lesions, assess disease severity and gather valuable clinical information to guide diagnostic and therapeutic decisions. Early recognition and diagnosis of psoriasis are crucial for initiating timely interventions and improving outcomes for affected individuals.

MANAGEMENT

The management and treatment of psoriasis involves a multidisciplinary approach with the aim of reducing inflammation, controlling symptoms, preventing flare-ups and improving quality of life. Treatment strategies vary depending on the severity of the condition, its impact on the patient's life and individual preferences. There are a broad range of treatments available for psoriasis, and management strategies can be effective. As psoriasis is unique to each individual, determining the right treatment or combination of treatments will often entail an exploratory and refined approach.

In the primary care setting, treatment is usually overseen by a general practice nurse or general practitioner. Initially, psoriasis management often commences with topical therapies, available in various formulations (such as creams, ointments and gels) containing a range of active ingredients. Topical therapies are often the first-line treatment for mild-to-moderate psoriasis. Table 3.3 discusses some of the main topical treatments.

If psoriasis is severe or if the various types of topical treatments are not working, the patient is referred to a dermatologist. There are a range of treatments available from a dermatologist. UV light therapy reduces inflammation in the skin and can be effective for psoriasis and other inflammatory skin conditions. Both narrowband UVB and psoralen plus ultraviolet A (PUVA) therapy have been shown to be effective in treating psoriasis by suppressing inflammation and reducing abnormal skin cell growth.

Systemic treatments affect the entire body rather than targeting just one area, as is the case with topical therapy or UV therapy. These treatments are reserved for moderate-to-severe psoriasis, which has not successfully responded to topical treatments or UV therapy or for those who cannot have more UV therapy. In the UK, the most commonly used systemic treatments are:

- Methotrexate

- Ciclosporin

- Acitretin

Biologic medications are specifically designed to mimic chemicals that are naturally found within the body and act to correct something that is going wrong. These medications aim to address abnormalities or dysfunctions within the body by mimicking the actions of specific chemicals. Essentially, biologics work to restore balance or correct imbalances in biological processes by acting as substitutes for natural compounds.

These medications are designed to target and block specific immune system molecules involved in the inflammatory process of psoriasis. They are administered via injection or infusion and are usually reserved for patients with moderate-to-severe psoriasis who have not responded to other treatments or have contraindications to conventional systemic therapies. NICE (2017) has issued guidelines for when biologics can be prescribed.

Lifestyle changes can help to manage psoriasis and improve overall well-being. These may include maintaining a healthy diet, managing stress levels, avoiding triggers such as smoking or excessive alcohol consumption and practising good skin care habits. Patient education plays

Table 3.3   Some topical treatment options

Topical treatment	Discussion
Moisturisers and emollients	Moisturisers make the skin much more comfortable, decreasing dryness, scaling, cracking and soreness and itching.
	They may allow the other active treatments being used such as coal tar or vitamin D to be better absorbed.
	Emollient therapy often refers to the use of soap substitutes and bath oils, as well as the application of creams or ointments. Moisturisers typically refer to the creams and ointments themselves.
Vitamin D derivatives	Topical vitamin D treatments are often one of the first topical treatments to be prescribed to people with psoriasis. Topical vitamin D treatments can come in ointment, lotion, gel and foam formations.
	These treatments act by slowing down the production of skin cells and have an anti-inflammatory effect. This leads to an improvement in psoriasis symptoms for some people.
	Topical vitamin D treatments can be used separately or in combination with topical steroid treatments.
Topical steroids	This is a treatment option for people whose psoriasis covers only a small amount of their body. They should not be used on more widespread psoriasis. They may be used separately or in combination with topical vitamin D treatments.
	Topical steroids can also be used to treat psoriasis in sensitive areas such as the face, genitals and skin folds. Less-potent steroids (mild or moderately potent) are usually used in the sensitive areas and for a shorter length of time, for example, two weeks rather than four.
Coal tar preparations	This is a thick, heavy oil that is thought to have anti-inflammatory and anti-scaling properties useful in the treatment of plaque psoriasis. The treatments are topical and come in lotion, cream, ointment, shampoo and bath additive forms.
Calcineurin inhibitors	Calcineurin inhibitors are similar in action to topical steroids. They reduce inflammation but do not have the same side effects. They may be more appropriate for longer-term use or in sensitive areas.

Source: Adapted from Psoriasis Association (2023).

a crucial role in psoriasis management. Patients are offered information and advice about their condition, treatment options and self-care measures. Support groups and resources can also provide valuable emotional support and practical advice for coping with psoriasis.

PSYCHOLOGICAL SUPPORT

Individuals respond differently to life events, making it essential to inquire about how psoriasis affects their daily lives. This impact may manifest in various ways, such as avoiding situations where skin exposure is necessary, leading to physical health consequences such as cardiovascular disease and obesity due to unhealthy lifestyle choices. Some people may resort to concealing their skin with excessive clothing or avoid intimacy with their partners. In cases where emotional and psychological challenges are prominent, a referral to a clinical psychologist may be beneficial (Peters 2019). Working collaboratively with patients, psychologists can address body image concerns, issues related to sexuality, quality of life and develop personalised coping strategies. These aspects are integral considerations in psoriasis management and effective counselling can complement therapeutic interventions.

The management and treatment of psoriasis requires a personalised approach that considers the severity of the condition, patient preferences and treatment goals. Implementing a comprehensive treatment plan that combines topical therapies, phototherapy, systemic medications, lifestyle modifications and patient information has the potential to effectively control symptoms, minimise flare-ups and improve the quality of life for individuals living with psoriasis.

HEALTH TEACHING

Health teaching focuses on reducing trigger factors for the exacerbation of psoriasis and encouraging the patient to apply the topical therapies and attend for phototherapy. Keeping the skin soft and moist can offer comfort as well as avoid itching and the use of irritating cosmetics and soap (Stephens 2022).

Patients are offered information and advice about the nature of psoriasis as a chronic inflammatory skin condition, which includes its causes, triggers and potential complications. Information is provided about the different types of psoriasis and their characteristic features. The various treatment modalities available for psoriasis are discussed with the patient including topical therapies, phototherapy, systemic medications and biological agents. An explanation is provided concerning the benefits, risks and potential side effects of each treatment option, as well as the importance of adherence to prescribed regimens.

Skin care techniques are discussed with patients to help manage psoriasis symptoms and prevent flare-ups. This may include recommendations for gentle cleansing, moisturising and avoiding irritants or harsh chemicals that can exacerbate skin inflammation.

The patient is encouraged to adopt healthy lifestyle habits that can positively impact their psoriasis, such as maintaining a balanced diet, managing stress, getting regular exercise, stopping smoking and limiting alcohol consumption. Emphasise the role of lifestyle factors in reducing inflammation and improving overall health.

Strategies for coping with stress are suggested, as stress can trigger or exacerbate psoriasis flare-ups in some individuals. Techniques such as mindfulness, relaxation exercises and cognitive-behavioural therapy may be helpful in managing stress and promoting emotional well-being.

Patients are advised about the importance of sun protection, as sunburn can trigger psoriasis flare-ups. The use of broad-spectrum sunscreen, protective clothing and seeking shade during peak sunlight hours is recommended.

Potential complications associated with psoriasis, such as psoriatic arthritis, cardiovascular disease and metabolic syndrome, are highlighted. The signs and symptoms of these complications are outlined and the importance of regular monitoring and follow-up emphasised.

The support resources available to individuals with psoriasis, such as patient advocacy groups, online forums and educational materials, are provided. Patients are encouraged to consider support networks where they can connect with others living with psoriasis and share experiences and advice.

Addressing these health teaching needs can empower individuals with psoriasis to take an active role in managing their condition, making informed decisions about treatment options and improving their overall quality of life.

CONCLUSION

Psoriasis is a complex, inflammatory skin condition that significantly impacts the quality of life of affected individuals. It is characterised by well-defined, red papules and plaques that are covered with silvery scales. Various factors contribute to psoriasis, including genetics and common triggers such as trauma, infection and certain medications. Symptoms typically include minimal to severe itching, with significant cosmetic implications that may require emotional and psychological support. Psoriatic arthritis affects some individuals; the condition can affect any joint in the body and commonly involves the fingers, toes, wrists, knees and ankles. It may also cause inflammation in other tissues, such as the tendons and ligaments and can lead to complications such as joint damage and deformities if left untreated. Diagnosis of psoriasis relies on the appearance and distribution of lesions along with a detailed medical history. Treatment options encompass topical therapies, phototherapy and systemic medications for severe cases.

GLOSSARY OF TERMS

Biologics: Medications derived from living organisms that target specific components of the immune system involved in psoriasis inflammation.

Calcineurin inhibitors: Topical medications that suppress immune system activity and reduce inflammation in psoriasis.

Coal tar preparations: Topical treatments containing coal tar, which can help reduce inflammation, itching and scaling associated with psoriasis.

Cyclosporine: An oral immunosuppressant medication used to treat severe psoriasis by suppressing the immune system's overactivity.

Guttate psoriasis: A type of psoriasis characterised by small, droplet-shaped lesions that often develop suddenly, typically triggered by infections such as streptococcal throat infections.

Koebner phenomenon: The development of new psoriatic lesions at sites of skin injury or trauma, such as cuts, scrapes or surgical scars.

Methotrexate: An oral medication that suppresses the immune system and reduces inflammation, often used to treat moderate to severe psoriasis.

Phototherapy: Treatment involving exposure to ultraviolet (UV) light, which can help reduce inflammation and slow the growth of skin cells in psoriasis.

Plaque psoriasis: The most common form of psoriasis, characterised by well-defined, raised red patches covered with silvery-white scales.

Psoriasis Area and Severity Index: A numerical scale used to assess the severity of psoriasis based on the extent of skin involvement, erythema (redness), induration (thickness) and scaling.

Psoriatic arthritis: A form of arthritis that affects some individuals with psoriasis, characterised by joint inflammation, pain, swelling and stiffness.

Systemic medications: Oral or injectable medications that work throughout the body to treat psoriasis, including methotrexate, cyclosporine and biological agents.

Topical treatments: Medications applied directly to the skin to treat psoriasis, including corticosteroids, vitamin D analogues, coal tar preparations and calcineurin inhibitors.

UV light therapy: Phototherapy involving exposure to UV light, which can help reduce inflammation and slow the growth of skin cells in psoriasis.

Vitamin D analogues: Synthetic forms of vitamin D that can help regulate skin cell growth and reduce inflammation in psoriasis when applied topically.

MULTIPLE CHOICE QUESTIONS

1. Which of the following is the most common form of psoriasis?
   a) Guttate psoriasis
   b) Plaque psoriasis
   c) Pustular psoriasis
   d) Inverse psoriasis

2. What is the primary goal of treatment for psoriasis?
   a) Complete cure
   b) Symptom relief
   c) Prevention of flare-ups
   d) Prevention of psoriatic arthritis

3. Which class of medications works by suppressing the immune system's overactivity in psoriasis?
   a) Corticosteroids
   b) Topical calcineurin inhibitors
   c) Biologics
   d) Vitamin D analogues

4. What is the recommended first-line treatment for mild-to-moderate plaque psoriasis?
   a) Methotrexate
   b) Topical corticosteroids
   c) Cyclosporine
   d) Biological agents

5. Which vitamin plays a role in regulating skin cell growth and may be used in topical treatment for psoriasis?
   a) Vitamin A
   b) Vitamin C
   c) Vitamin D
   d) Vitamin E

6. What is the primary advantage of biologic medications in treating psoriasis?
   a) Low cost
   b) Oral administration
   c) Long-term safety profile
   d) Targeted mechanism of action

7. Which of the following is a potential complication of untreated psoriasis?
   a) Psoriatic arthritis
   b) Cardiovascular disease
   c) Metabolic syndrome
   d) All of the above

8. What is the term for the small, pinpoint bleeding that occurs when adherent psoriatic scales are scraped off?
   a) Koebner phenomenon
   b) Munro's microabscesses
   c) Auspitz sign
   d) Parakeratosis

9. Which topical treatment for psoriasis should be used cautiously in sensitive areas such as the face, groin and armpits due to its potential for skin thinning?
    a) Coal tar preparations
    b) Topical corticosteroids
    c) Vitamin D analogues
    d) Calcineurin inhibitors

10. Which of the following is NOT a common trigger for psoriasis flare-ups?
    a) Stress
    b) Infections
    c) Cold weather
    d) Medications

REFERENCES

Castro, L. (2019). Skin disorders (Chapter 26). In: *Learning to Care* (ed. I. Peate). London: Elsevier.

Chowdhury, M.U., Katugampola, R.P., and Finlay, A.Y. (2019). *Dermatology at a Glance*, 2e. Oxford: Wiley.

Feldman, S.R. and Kruege, G.G. (2005). Psoriasis assessment tools in clinical trials. *Annals of the Rheumatic Disease* 64 (Suppl II): ii65–ii68. doi: 10.1136/ard.2004.031237.

Griffiths, C.E., Armstrong, A.W., Gudjonsson, J.E. et al. (2021). Psoriasis. *Lancet* 397: 1301–1315. doi: 10.1016/S0140-6736(20)32549-6.

Hagler, D., Harding, M.M., Kwong, J. et al. (2023). *Lewis's Medical-Surgical Nursing*. St Louis: Elsevier.

Johnson, M.A. and Armstrong, A.W. (2013). Clinical and histologic diagnostic guidelines for psoriasis: a critical review. *Clinical Reviews in Allergy and Immunology* 44 (2): 166–172.

Kamiya, K., Kishimoto, M., Sugai, J. et al. (2019). Risk factors for the development of psoriasis. *International Journal of Molecular Science* 20 (18): 4347. doi: 10.3390/ijms20184347.

Mattessich, S. and Grant-Kels, J.M. (2020). Ethical aspects of the use of photography in clinical medicine (Chapter 5). In: *Photography in Clinical Medicine* (ed. P. Pasquali). Berlin: Springer.

National Institute for Health and Care Excellence (2017). Psoriasis: assessment and management. https://www.nice.org.uk/guidance/cg153/resourc es/psoriasis-assessment-and-management-pdf-35 109629621701 (accessed May 2024).

National Psoriasis Foundation (2022). Causes and triggers. https://www.psoriasis.org/causes/ (accessed May 2024).

National Psoriasis Foundation (2024). Plaque psoriasis. https://www.psoriasis.org/plaque/ (accessed May 2024).

Peters, J. (2019). Nursing patients with skin disorders (Chapter 13). In: *Alexander's Nursing Practice*, 5e (ed. I. Peate). London: Elsevier.

Primary Care Dermatology Society (2023). What is psoriasis? https://www.pcds.org.uk/files/pils/ Psoriasis-PIL-Dec-23-for-PDF.pdf (accessed May 2024).

Psoriasis Association (2023). About psoriasis. https:// www.psoriasis-association.org.uk/about-psoriasis (accessed May 2024).

Stephens, M. (2022). The person with a skin disorder (Chapter 35). In: *Nursing Practice*, 3e (ed. I. Peate and A. Mitchell). Oxford: Wiley.

The word 'eczema' originates from the Greek word 'ekzema', which means 'to boil over' or 'to break out'. This term accurately reflects the characteristic symptoms of eczema, which involves the skin breaking out in patches of inflammation and irritation.

Eczema is also known as atopic dermatitis and neurodermatitis (International League of Dermatological Societies [ILDS] 2022). This is a common skin condition, a non-communicable condition that is characterised by inflammation, redness, itching and sometimes blistering or oozing of the skin. Eczema often appears as patches of dry, scaly skin that can be itchy and uncomfortable; it can vary in severity from mild to severe and can affect people of all ages. It is most common in infants and young children. While the exact cause of eczema is not fully understood, it is believed to involve a combination of genetic, environmental and immune system factors. Treatment aims to reduce inflammation and itching.

TYPES OF DERMATITIS

There are several types, including atopic dermatitis. Eczema encompasses a range of skin conditions marked by inflammation, itchiness, redness and occasional blistering or skin fissures.

ATOPIC DERMATITIS

The term atopic refers to a collection of conditions that include eczema, asthma, hay fever and food allergies. What unites these conditions is that they all involve an immune system response with heightened allergic activity. Individuals with atopic conditions tend to have immune systems that react more strongly to allergens compared to those without these conditions.

Atopic dermatitis is the most common form of eczema and often begins in infancy or childhood (Stephens 2022). It tends to run in families with a history of asthma, hay fever or other allergies. Symptoms include dry, itchy and inflamed skin, often occurring on the face, scalp, hands and feet. Flare-ups can be triggered by factors such as irritants, allergens, stress and climate changes.

CONTACT DERMATITIS

Contact dermatitis occurs when the skin comes into contact with an irritant or allergen, leading to redness, itching and inflammation. Irritant contact dermatitis is more common and is caused by substances such as soaps, detergents and chemicals. Allergic contact dermatitis occurs when the skin develops an allergic reaction to a specific substance, such as metals, fragrances or latex.

This common skin condition occurs when the skin comes into contact with substances that either irritate the skin or trigger an allergic reaction. There are two main types: irritant contact dermatitis and allergic contact dermatitis.

IRRITANT CONTACT DERMATITIS

This form of contact dermatitis is more prevalent and is caused by direct contact with substances that damage or irritate the skin. It can result from exposure to a wide range of substances, including soaps, detergents, solvents, acids, alkalis and certain plants. Symptoms usually include redness, itching, burning and inflammation of the skin at the site of contact. The severity of irritant contact dermatitis can vary depending on factors such as the strength and duration of exposure to the irritant, as well as individual skin sensitivity.

ALLERGIC CONTACT DERMATITIS

Allergic contact dermatitis occurs when the immune system reacts to a specific substance (known as an allergen) as though it were harmful, triggering an allergic response. Common allergens that can cause allergic contact dermatitis include metals found in jewellery, fragrances (in perfumes, cosmetics and personal care products), preservatives, latex (found in gloves and certain medical products) and certain medications. Symptoms of allergic contact dermatitis can include redness, itching, swelling and the development of a rash or blisters at the site of contact.

Unlike irritant contact dermatitis, allergic contact dermatitis requires prior sensitisation to the allergen, meaning that initial exposure does not typically cause a reaction. However, subsequent exposures can lead to an allergic response.

Both types of contact dermatitis can cause discomfort and may require treatment to alleviate symptoms and promote healing. Treatment may involve:

- Avoiding the triggering substances (if possible).

- Using topical corticosteroids or anti-inflammatory creams to reduce inflammation and itching.

- Applying moisturisers to help repair the skin barrier.

- Taking oral antihistamines to relieve itching (especially in cases of allergic contact dermatitis).

- In severe cases, stronger medications are required or patch testing may be recommended to identify specific allergens.

See Table 4.1 on contact dermatitis related to health and care workers.

Table 4.1 Contact dermatitis related to health and care workers

Irritant contact dermatitis:

Health and care workers frequently use hand hygiene products such as soap and hand sanitisers to prevent the spread of infection. However, frequent handwashing and exposure to alcohol-based sanitisers can reduce the skin's natural oils, leading to irritation and dryness.

Cleaning agents, disinfectants and chemicals used for surface disinfection can also irritate the skin, especially if corrective protective measures such as gloves are not used consistently.

Prolonged or repeated exposure to irritants can compromise the skin barrier, making it more susceptible to irritation and inflammation.

Allergic contact dermatitis:

Health and care workers may develop allergic contact dermatitis in response to specific allergens commonly found in the care settings. Latex allergy, for example, is a well-known concern among care workers; latex gloves are frequently used in patient care. Other potential allergens encountered include certain medications (e.g. antibiotics, antiseptics), adhesive tapes, dressings and various chemicals used in medical procedures.

Allergic contact dermatitis can develop gradually over time, as health and care workers become sensitised to specific allergens through repeated exposure. Once sensitisation occurs, even minimal contact with the allergen can trigger an allergic reaction.

SEBORRHOEIC DERMATITIS

Seborrhoeic dermatitis primarily affects areas of the skin with high oil production, such as the scalp, face (especially around the eyebrows, nose and ears) and upper chest. It is characterised by redness, greasy or flaky yellow scales and itching. Seborrhoeic dermatitis may be exacerbated by factors including stress, hormones and certain medical conditions.

POMPHOLYX ECZEMA

Pompholyx eczema is also known as dyshidrotic eczema. This typically affects the palms of the hands, soles of the feet and sides of the fingers. It is characterised by small, itchy blisters that can be painful and may lead to peeling, cracking and swelling of the skin. The exact cause is unknown, but factors such as stress, allergies and exposure to irritants may contribute to flare-ups.

NUMMULAR ECZEMA

Nummular eczema is seen as coin-shaped patches of red, inflamed skin that may ooze, crust or scale. These patches can be itchy and are often found on the arms, legs, back and torso. The cause of nummular eczema is not fully understood, but it may be triggered by factors such as dry skin, cold weather and certain skin injuries.

VENOUS ECZEMA

Venous eczema also known as stasis dermatitis or gravitational dermatitis occurs in the lower legs and ankles due to poor circulation caused by venous insufficiency. Symptoms include redness, swelling, itching and sometimes ulceration of the skin. Venous dermatitis is more common in older adults and individuals with conditions such as varicose veins and obesity.

Each type of eczema may have specific triggers and treatment approaches. This chapter will focus on atopic dermatitis.

PATHOPHYSIOLOGICAL CHANGES ASSOCIATED WITH ATOPIC DERMATITIS

Although the exact cause of eczema remains unknown, it is thought to be the result of a combination of genetic predisposition and environmental influences (Kim, Kim, and Leung 2019).

Atopic dermatitis is the most prevalent chronic inflammatory skin condition and can have a substantial impact on quality of life (Teasdale et al. 2021). Genetic predisposition, disruption of the epidermal barrier and immune system dysregulation are key elements in this condition. A compromised skin barrier may serve as the initial phase in the progression of the atopic march and atopic dermatitis, leading to subsequent skin inflammation and allergic sensitisation.

A protein called filaggrin is essential for maintaining the pH balance and moisture levels in the skin, particularly within the stratum corneum (the outermost layer of the skin, see Chapter 1 of this book). Filaggrin is essential for the structural integrity of the stratum corneum. When filaggrin breaks down, it produces smaller molecules that are also important for the skin's barrier function. In individuals with atopic dermatitis, who have deficient filaggrin, there is an increased permeability of the stratum corneum due to abnormalities in the structure of the cells in the stratum corneum, leading to impaired barrier function.

Atopic march is a term used to describe the progression of allergic diseases. Yang, Fu, and Zhou (2020) report that there is a sequential progression of allergies, typically starting with skin-related conditions before affecting the digestive and respiratory systems. Initially, manifestations include atopic dermatitis (eczema) and food allergies during infancy, followed by the development of allergic asthma and allergic rhinitis (nasal allergies) in childhood. See Figure 4.1 on atopic dermatitis and associated conditions.

Certain immune system molecules, specifically type 2 cytokines, interleukin-17 and interleukin-22, play a role in damaging the skin's protective barrier and initiating the development of atopic dermatitis. These molecules contribute to the dysfunction of the skin barrier, which is a key characteristic of atopic dermatitis. Understanding and targeting these immune molecules may be important in developing therapies for the prevention and treatment of atopic dermatitis.

Novel therapeutic approaches are centred on enhancing skin barrier integrity and addressing specific immune pathways implicated in atopic dermatitis. A deeper understanding of atopic dermatitis pathophysiology will pave the way for a more tailored precision approach to both prevention and treatment.

Understanding the pathophysiological changes that are associated with atopic dermatitis is essential for developing targeted therapies that are aimed at restoring skin barrier function (a compromised skin barrier is one of the hallmark features of atopic dermatitis), modulating immune responses and alleviating symptoms such as itching and inflammation.

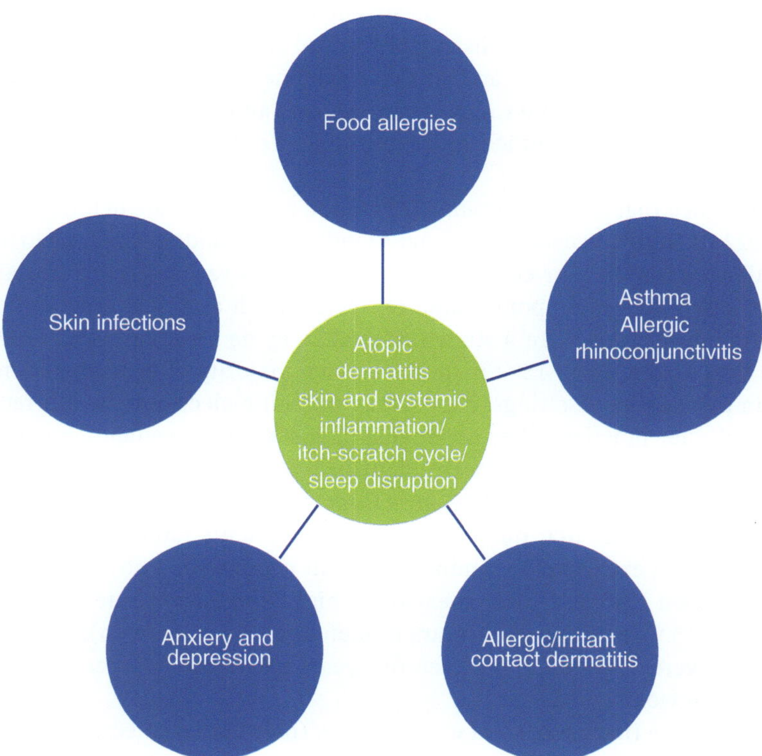

FIGURE 4.1 Atopic dermatitis and associated conditions. *Source:* Adapted from ILDS (2022).

Additionally, addressing environmental triggers and lifestyle factors can play a crucial role in managing the condition effectively.

EPIDEMIOLOGY

Atopic dermatitis brings with it the most significant burden among all skin conditions. It represents an important global public health concern (ILDS 2022). The prevalence of this common condition is increasing (Yang, Fu, and Zhou 2020). Understanding the epidemiology and demographics of atopic dermatitis is important for several reasons. The epidemiological data help assess the burden of atopic dermatitis within populations, providing estimates of how many individuals are affected. This information is essential for healthcare planning, resource allocation and prioritising public health interventions.

Understanding the distribution of atopic eczema across different demographic groups can help to tailor services to meet the specific needs of affected populations. This may include specialised clinics, educational programmes and support services for individuals with atopic dermatitis. Epidemiological data guide research priorities by highlighting gaps in knowledge and areas that require further investigation. For example, identifying disparities in atopic dermatitis prevalence among groups may prompt research into genetic and environmental factors underlying these differences.

Determining prevalence presents difficulties due to the fluctuating nature of atopic eczema, with studies often concentrating on the occurrence of active symptoms. Incidence rates in children change based on age and gender, while data for both adults and children are confounded by inaccurate or incomplete documentation of eczema diagnosis and treatment in primary healthcare settings. Establishing prevalence is challenging because atopic eczema is a remitting–relapsing condition and studies sometimes focus on the incidence of active eczema. The incidence in children varies according to age and sex and data for both adults and children is limited by inaccurate/incomplete recording of eczema diagnosis and management in primary care.

It is estimated that there are around 223 million people who are living with atopic dermatitis in 2022 (ILDS 2022), of which around 43 million are children aged one to four years.

Prevalence estimates for eczema exhibit significant variability, particularly among adults, with a lack of contemporary data on factors such as urban environments influencing eczema development. In a study undertaken by de Lusignan et al. (2020), prevalence rates range from 2.5 to 15% in adults. Since a majority of eczema patients receive treatment in primary care settings, databases containing electronic health records from general practitioner practices offer a valuable data source for epidemiological analyses; approximately 500 000 individuals were identified as having eczema between 1998 and 2015, equating to a prevalence of 10%. It is important to note that this study primarily aimed to assess cardiovascular outcomes in eczema patients rather than focusing solely on prevalence, and it exclusively examined the adult population. The incidence of eczema in children between 1997 and 2015 revealed the highest incidence rates in those younger than two years (15.9 per 100 person-years in men and 11.7 in women), while the lowest incidence rates were observed in children five years and above (0.4 per 100 person-years in men and 0.5 in women).

The occurrence (incidence) and existing cases (prevalence) of eczema reported by de Lusignan et al. (2020) showed a bimodal age distribution pattern. The highest incidence of eczema was observed in children under the age of one year, with an incidence rate of 15.0

cases per 100 person-years. This incidence rate gradually decreased during childhood and early adulthood, followed by a gradual increase after the age of 50 years. Additionally, the study identified notable differences in the occurrence and prevalence of eczema based on factors such as gender, socioeconomic status, ethnicity and geographical location.

Understanding the epidemiological and demographic characteristics of atopic dermatitis is essential for identifying at-risk populations, guiding preventive strategies and improving healthcare resource allocation. Furthermore, ongoing research into the environmental and genetic determinants of atopic dermatitis may lead to more targeted approaches for disease management and prevention in the future.

RISK FACTORS

Atopic dermatitis is a complex condition with causes that are not yet fully understood. It results from a complex interplay of genetic, environmental and immunological factors. Environmental factors (where a person lives and what irritants they are exposed to), genetics and having an overactive immune system are all believed to play a role in developing atopic dermatitis. Risk factors include a family history of atopic dermatitis or allergies, high levels of stress and extremely dry skin.

Filaggrin deficiency is associated with an early onset of atopic dermatitis. Alterations or changes (mutations) in the filaggrin gene can lead to a decrease in the production of filaggrin protein. This reduction in filaggrin production can weaken or impair the function of the skin's barrier. As a result, the skin becomes more vulnerable to external irritants, allergens and microbes, which can contribute to atopic dermatitis (Hadi et al. 2021). Table 4.2 outlines the risk factors associated with atopic dermatitis.

Table 4.2 Risk factors associated with atopic dermatitis

Risk factor	Discussion
Genetics	Atopic dermatitis often runs in families, suggesting a strong genetic predisposition. Specific gene variations, particularly mutations in the filaggrin gene, have been linked to impaired skin barrier function, which is a hallmark feature of atopic dermatitis. Individuals with a family history of eczema, asthma or allergic rhinitis are at higher risk of developing atopic dermatitis.
Immune dysregulation	Atopic dermatitis is characterised by immune dysregulation. The dysregulation of the immune system results in increased production of pro-inflammatory cytokines and IgE antibodies, which promote chronic inflammation and allergic responses in the skin, contributing to symptoms of atopic dermatitis.
Skin barrier dysfunction	Disruptions in the epidermal barrier allow irritants, allergens and microorganisms to penetrate the skin more easily, triggering inflammatory responses and exacerbating eczema symptoms.
Environmental factors	Various environmental factors can influence the development and exacerbation of atopic dermatitis. Exposure to allergens, such as pollen, dust mites, pet dander and certain foods, can trigger allergic reactions and eczema flare-ups in susceptible individuals. Additionally, irritants such as harsh soaps, detergents and chemicals can further compromise the skin barrier and worsen eczema symptoms.

(Continued)

Table 4.2 (*Continued*)

Risk factor	Discussion
Climate	Climate and weather conditions can impact atopic dermatitis symptoms. Dry, cold weather can exacerbate skin dryness and irritation, leading to increased itchiness and eczema flare-ups. Conversely, hot and humid weather can promote sweating and friction, aggravating skin inflammation and discomfort in individuals with atopic dermatitis.
Microbial factors	Microbial colonisation of the skin, particularly by *Staphylococcus aureus* bacteria, is commonly observed in individuals with atopic dermatitis. The overgrowth of bacteria on the skin can exacerbate inflammation, impair skin barrier function and contribute to recurrent skin infections in eczema patients.
Allergic sensitisation	Individuals with atopic dermatitis often have heightened immune responses to allergens, leading to allergic sensitisation and allergic reactions. Food allergies, in particular, are common in children with atopic dermatitis, although not all cases of eczema are triggered by food allergies.
Psychological factors	Psychological stress and emotional factors can influence the severity and course of atopic dermatitis. Stress can exacerbate inflammation, trigger itchiness and impair skin barrier function, leading to increased eczema symptoms. Conversely, eczema symptoms themselves can cause significant psychological distress, impacting the quality of life and mental well-being.
Lifestyle factors	Certain lifestyle factors, such as smoking, obesity and inadequate skincare practices, can increase the risk and severity of atopic dermatitis. Smoking has been associated with worsened eczema symptoms and impaired treatment response, while obesity is linked to chronic inflammation and metabolic dysregulation, which can exacerbate atopic dermatitis.
Medical history	Individuals with a history of other allergic conditions, such as asthma, allergic rhinitis or allergic conjunctivitis, are more likely to develop atopic dermatitis. Additionally, certain medical conditions, such as immunodeficiency disorders or autoimmune diseases, may predispose individuals to eczema or exacerbate existing symptoms.
Hormonal changes in women	Hormonal fluctuations in women can influence the course of atopic dermatitis. Some women with atopic dermatitis may experience worsening of symptoms, such as increased itching, redness and inflammation, in the days leading up to menstruation. This phenomenon is often referred to as premenstrual flare-ups. Hormonal changes, particularly fluctuations in oestrogen and progesterone levels during the menstrual cycle, are thought to contribute to these exacerbations. Pregnancy can also impact the severity of atopic dermatitis symptoms for some women. While pregnancy can lead to improvement in atopic dermatitis symptoms for some individuals, others may experience worsening or onset of atopic dermatitis during pregnancy. Hormonal changes, immune alterations and stress associated with pregnancy are believed to influence the course of atopic dermatitis during this time.

Source: Adapted from American Academy of Dermatology Association (2023), Hadi et al. (2021) and Hale et al. (2019).

Having an awareness and understanding of the risk factors associated with atopic dermatitis is essential for prevention, early identification, improved treatment outcomes, public health strategies, research and resource allocation, ultimately leading to improved outcomes for individuals and families affected by the condition.

CLINICAL PRESENTATION

The clinical presentation of atopic dermatitis can vary widely among individuals and may change over time. The hallmark symptom of atopic dermatitis is a red, itchy rash, often referred to as eczema. This rash typically appears in characteristic locations, including the flexural areas (such as the elbows, knees and neck), as well as the face, hands and feet. The skin lesions that are associated with atopic dermatitis are characterised by papules, oozing vesicles on red swollen skin (although redness is more difficult to determine in darker skin and may not always be apparent), crusting and scaling.

Intense pruritus is a key feature and a predominant symptom of atopic dermatitis and can be intense and distressing, leading to scratching and further skin damage. The intensity of itch experienced may result in repeated scratching of the skin in order to relieve the itch. This often leads to more skin damage and then more itch, the itch–scratch–itch cycle (ILDS 2022; see Figure 4.2). The itchiness associated with atopic dermatitis often worsens at night and this can disrupt sleep and impact the quality of life.

Symptoms of atopic dermatitis may worsen or flare-up in response to certain triggers, including exposure to allergens, irritants, environmental factors, stress, sweating and certain foods.

Chronic scratching and rubbing of the skin can lead to lichenification, a thickening and hardening of the skin. Additionally, repeated inflammation and scratching can cause secondary changes such as excoriation (scratch marks), fissures (cracks) and erosions (open sores).

The distribution of atopic dermatitis lesions may vary depending on the age of the individual. In infants and young children, the rash often appears on the face, scalp and extensor surfaces of the limbs. In adolescents and adults, the rash may localise to the flexural areas and hands.

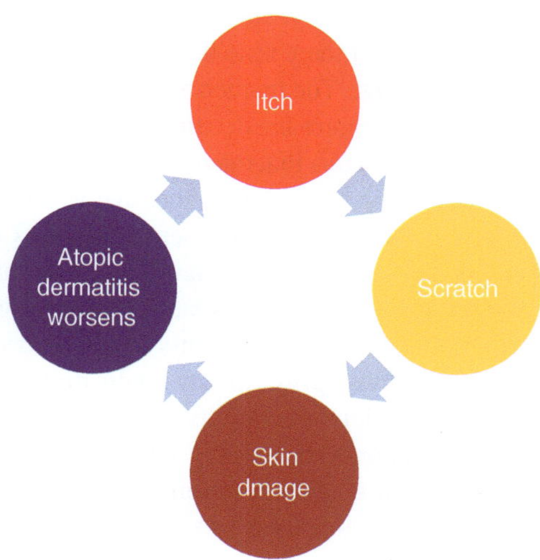

FIGURE 4.2 The itch–scratch–itch cycle

Atopic dermatitis is frequently associated with other allergic conditions, such as asthma, allergic rhinitis and food allergies. Individuals with atopic dermatitis may also have a personal or family history of these conditions.

Presentations can vary across different geographical areas. For instance, in Africa, there are reports of a higher prevalence of thickened and raised skin (papular lichenoid lesions), while in Southeast Asia, oozing lesions (exudative) are more frequently observed, often indicating bacterial skin infections. In India and Southeast Asia, lichenification and changes in skin colouration (hypo- or hyperpigmentation) are also common characteristics among patients with atopic dermatitis (ILDS 2022).

CLINICAL INVESTIGATIONS AND DIAGNOSIS

Diagnosis of atopic dermatitis is clinical and is made from the presentation and patient's history (Peters 2019). Atopic dermatitis is sometimes difficult to differentiate from other dermatoses. The diagnosis of atopic dermatitis depends on excluding other conditions. There is a need to obtain a detailed medical history, perform a physical examination and instigate other tests and investigations depending on individual patient needs.

HISTORY TAKING

Information from the patient (or parents/carers) about their medical background, symptoms and any relevant factors related to their condition involves several steps. The process begins by establishing a rapport with the patient and conducting a structured interview. During the consultation, the patient is asked open-ended questions; this can encourage the patient to provide relevant information about their symptoms, past medical history and family history of allergic conditions. Probing questions are also used to explore specific aspects of their medical history related to atopic dermatitis.

Inquiries are made about the patient's symptoms onset, duration and progression of symptoms related to atopic dermatitis. Understanding when the symptoms of atopic dermatitis first appeared, how long they have been present and how they have progressed over time provide valuable insights into the nature and severity of the disease. Ask the patient to describe their typical symptoms, including itching, redness, dryness, scaling and any associated discomfort; the diagnosis is unlikely to be atopic eczema if there is no itch (National Institute for Health and Care Excellence [NICE] 2007), regardless of age. The frequency and severity of flare-ups, as well as any factors that worsen or alleviate their symptoms are documented.

Potential triggers or exacerbating factors that may contribute to flare-ups of atopic dermatitis are explored with the patient. Identifying triggers or factors that worsen atopic dermatitis symptoms is important for developing personalised management strategies. Common triggers include allergens (such as dust mites, pet dander or pollen), irritants (such as harsh soaps or detergents), environmental factors (such as dry air or extreme temperatures), stress, sweating and certain foods.

The patient is asked about any previous treatments they have tried for atopic dermatitis, including over-the-counter medications, prescription medications, topical treatments and alternative therapies. A history of previous treatments for atopic dermatitis provides valuable information about the patient's response to therapy and helps guide future management decisions. It allows for an assessment of the effectiveness of prior interventions, to identify any adverse effects or treatment failures and tailor treatment plans based on individual patient responses. The patient is asked about their experiences with different treatments, including effectiveness, side effects and adherence to treatment regimens.

Atopic dermatitis has a strong genetic component and a family history of allergic conditions, such as atopic dermatitis, asthma, allergic rhinitis (hay fever) or food allergies, increases the risk of developing atopic dermatitis. Understanding the familial predisposition to allergic diseases helps assess the patient's overall risk profile and may influence treatment decisions and recommendations for preventive measures. Any known familial patterns of allergic diseases are documented and the person is asked about the severity and age of onset of these conditions in family members.

A discussion is conducted regarding any other relevant medical conditions or comorbidities that the patient may have, as well as any medications they are currently taking. The person is asked about symptoms of associated conditions such as asthma, allergic rhinitis, anxiety, depression or sleep disturbances, as these may impact the management of atopic dermatitis.

All the information that is obtained from the patient during the interview is documented in a structured format, such as a medical history form or electronic health record, and local policy and procedure is adhered to. Documentation is thorough, accurate and organised so that it can be accessed for future reference and decision-making.

PHYSICAL EXAMINATION

A thorough physical examination will be conducted to assess the skin's appearance and any associated symptoms. The procedure is explained to the patient (careers/family), consent is obtained, if appropriate, a chaperone should be offered and local policy and procedure regarding infection prevention and control adhered to. Privacy, dignity and comfort are maintained throughout.

The skin lesions are examined, and the distribution and severity of skin lesions are also evaluated, along with any signs of secondary infection or complications. The distribution and appearance of the rash will be influenced by the person's age, ethnicity, duration of the rash and the presence/absence of infection. Signs of excoriation may also be present. In adults, there is generalised dryness and itching, particularly with exposure to irritants. Eczema noted on the hands may be the primary manifestation.

In children and adults with long-standing disease, eczema is often localised to the flexure of the limbs. In infants, eczema primarily involves the face, the scalp and the extensor surfaces of the limbs. The nappy area is usually unaffected.

Acute eczema (flares) varies in appearance, from poorly demarcated redness to fluid in the skin (vesicles), scaling or crusting of the skin. Chronic eczema is characterised by thickened (lichenified) skin resulting from repeated scratching.

Follicular hyperkeratotic papules (keratosis pilaris; small, rough bumps on the skin's surface) that are typically asymptomatic may be present on the extensor surfaces of the upper arms, buttocks and anterior thighs. If eczema is weeping, crusted or there are pustules, with fever or malaise present, secondary bacterial infection should be considered.

INVESTIGATIONS

Investigations are rarely required to establish the diagnosis. Nevertheless, they can be beneficial in ruling out other potential conditions, particularly in individuals whose symptoms persist despite treatment. Laboratory investigations may include:

- Skin swabs: excoriated lesions may result in secondary infection.

- Skin scrapings: to exclude fungal infection.

- Skin biopsy: a small sample of skin tissue (biopsy) is taken for further examination using immunohistology techniques when there is uncertainty about the diagnosis. Immunohistology involves studying the tissue sample under a microscope to detect specific proteins or markers that may help confirm or clarify the diagnosis of a skin condition.

- Blood test: to ascertain the level of IgE (an immunoglobulin) or the presence of specific antibodies to external factors, e.g. house dust mite, pollen, cat/dog or food proteins.

Patch Testing This procedure might be performed to verify allergic contact dermatitis. Various patch tests can be conducted in which potential allergens such as nickel, fragrance, hair care products, plant materials and rubber are prepared in concentrations that typically elicit no reaction unless the patient is sensitive to them.

MANAGEMENT

The management of atopic dermatitis varies depending on the severity of the disease, the extent of skin involvement and the presence of any accompanying conditions (see Figure 4.1). Atopic dermatitis is a chronic, incurable but treatable skin disease (Stephens 2022).

Treatment usually follows a stepped-care approach, starting with the provision of patient education on avoiding irritants and triggers, as well as the correct application of topical therapies such as emollients and topical corticosteroids, which require correct guidance for effective use. In severe cases where topical therapies are insufficient, additional treatments such as phototherapy or systemic medications may be considered, although this decision is individualised based on factors such as the person's age, presence of other medical conditions, use of other medications, pregnancy status or prior treatments. Figure 4.3 provides an overview of the stepped approach.

Atopic dermatitis is a chronic condition and for some individuals, treatment may be needed long term. Treatment must be tailored to address the patient's most problematic symptoms at any given time, with the goal of improving quality of life and achieving life goals.

Providing care for individuals with atopic dermatitis extends beyond solely treating skin lesions. It should also encompass addressing associated health issues, such as allergic rhinitis and asthma. People with atopic dermatitis often experience additional conditions that include food

Severe	Continue with measures recommended below and select from them if appropriate		
	Various conventional systemic treatments		Various new systemic treatments
Moderate	Continue with measures recommended below and select from them if appropriate		
	Topical corticosteroids **PROACTIVE**	Topical calcineurin **PROACTIVE**	Phototherapy	Psychosomatic counselling
Mild	Continue with measures recommended below and select from them if appropriate		
	Topical corticosteroids **ACUTE**	Topical calcineurin inhibitors **REACTIVE**	Topical PDE4 inhibitors	Topical JAK inhibitors
Base line therapy	**Emollients**	**Avoiding allergens**	**Educational programmes**
	Daily, in sufficient quantity and adjust frequency to skin dryness	As much as possible in sensitised patients	Various responsive to need

FIGURE 4.3 A stepped approach

allergies, allergic and irritant contact dermatitis, decreased bone health and autoimmune diseases. These related health concerns should be taken into consideration when offering care and support to people with atopic dermatitis, viewing patients holistically rather than solely focusing on their skin condition (European Dermatology Forum 2022). This holistic approach also involves recognising the impact of atopic dermatitis on caregivers and family life. Shared decision-making principles guide treatment plans, incorporating patients' beliefs, lifestyles and preferences. Additionally, individuals with atopic dermatitis have a higher likelihood of developing mental health conditions such as anxiety and depression, experiencing suicidal ideation and facing challenges in daily life. It is therefore essential to implement psychological and educational interventions to positively influence disease progression and enhance overall psychological well-being.

See Table 4.3 for a discussion of the stepped approach to treating atopic dermatitis. This involves initiating treatment with basic measures and progressively advancing to more intensive interventions as needed. Treatment modalities are based on individual needs, local and national guidelines.

Table 4.3 A stepped approach to the treatment of atopic dermatitis

Approach	Discussion
Education and emollients	The first step involves patient education about atopic dermatitis and its management, including identifying triggers, proper skincare practices and the importance of moisturising. Emollients, such as moisturising creams or ointments, are recommended as the cornerstone of treatment to hydrate the skin and restore the damaged skin barrier. Patients are advised to use emollients regularly, especially after bathing, to lock in moisture.
Topical treatments	If emollients alone are insufficient to control symptoms, topical treatments may be added. Topical corticosteroids are commonly prescribed to reduce inflammation and itching in atopic dermatitis flare-ups. They are available in varying strengths and formulations and their use is tailored to the severity and location of symptoms. Topical calcineurin inhibitors, such as tacrolimus and pimecrolimus, are alternative options for patients who cannot tolerate or do not respond to corticosteroids.
Adjunctive therapies	In cases of moderate-to-severe atopic dermatitis or inadequate response to topical treatments, adjunctive therapies may be necessary. This may include phototherapy (light therapy), which involves exposing the skin to ultraviolet light under medical supervision. Phototherapy can help reduce inflammation and itching in atopic dermatitis lesions. Systemic medications, such as oral corticosteroids or immunosuppressants, may be considered for short-term use in severe cases or as maintenance therapy for chronic atopic dermatitis. However, these medications have potential side effects and require careful monitoring.
Specialist referral	If atopic dermatitis remains poorly controlled despite optimal treatment in primary care or if there are concerns about complications or comorbidities, referral to a dermatologist or allergy specialist may be warranted. Specialists can provide further evaluation, perform additional tests or procedures and offer advanced treatment options, including biological therapies for severe, refractory atopic dermatitis.

(Continued)

Table 4.3 (*Continued*)

Approach	Discussion
Maintenance and monitoring	Once symptoms are under control, maintenance therapy with emollients and intermittent use of topical treatments may be sufficient to prevent flare-ups and maintain remission. Regular follow-up visits are important to monitor disease activity, adjust treatment as needed and address any new concerns or complications.

Source: Adapted from ILDS (2022); NICE (2007).

The stepped approach to treating atopic dermatitis emphasises a gradual escalation of therapy based on disease severity and response to treatment, with the goal of achieving effective symptom control while minimising potential side effects and long-term complications. Collaboration between patients, caregivers and those who provide care and support to people is essential to tailor treatment plans to individual needs and improve outcomes for those with atopic dermatitis.

HEALTH TEACHING

Health teaching for individuals with atopic dermatitis is crucial for effective management. Patients and caregivers need to understand the nature of atopic dermatitis, including its triggers, symptoms and treatment options. Teaching should focus on proper skincare practices, such as gentle cleansing and regular moisturising to hydrate the skin and maintain the skin barrier. Patients should be educated on avoiding common triggers for atopic dermatitis flare-ups, including certain fabrics, harsh soaps, heat, sweat and stress. It is important to discuss strategies for managing itch, such as avoiding scratching and using cool compresses. Patients should be instructed on the correct use of topical treatments, including corticosteroids and calcineurin inhibitors, and encouraged to follow prescribed treatment regimens. Lifestyle modifications, including wearing loose-fitting clothing and stress management techniques, should be discussed. Patients should understand the importance of medication safety, including potential side effects and the need for regular follow-up appointments to monitor disease activity and adjust treatment as needed.

Emollients, including oils that are found in creams, lotions and ointments, can increase the flammability of fabrics and hair. Even after emollient products have dried, there remains a risk of fire when they come into contact with dressings, clothing, bedding or hair. Individuals using skincare or haircare products should exercise caution around open flames or lit cigarettes. It is advisable to launder clothing daily and change bed linens frequently if they have been in contact with emollients. However, even washing at high temperatures may not completely eliminate the risk of fire (Medicines and Healthcare Products Regulatory Agency 2021).

Offering comprehensive health education, information and advice, individuals with atopic dermatitis can gain a better understanding of their condition and develop the skills and knowledge needed to effectively manage their symptoms and improve their quality of life.

CONCLUSION

Atopic dermatitis presents a significant challenge for patients, caregivers and those who offer people care and support alike. This chronic inflammatory skin condition not only causes physical discomfort but can also have a profound impact on the psychological and emotional well-being of those affected. This chapter has explored the multifactorial nature of atopic dermatitis, including its complex pathophysiology, varied clinical presentation and the importance of individualised management strategies.

Effective management of atopic dermatitis requires a holistic approach that addresses both the acute symptoms and the underlying factors contributing to disease development and exacerbation. From patient education and skincare practices to pharmacological interventions and lifestyle modifications, there is a broad range of strategies available to help patients better manage their condition and improve their quality of life.

Working collaboratively with patients, their families and interdisciplinary care teams, there is the opportunity to improve care outcomes, reduce disease burden and empower individuals to lead healthier, more fulfilling lives despite the complexities of atopic dermatitis.

GLOSSARY OF TERMS

Allergen: Substance that triggers an allergic reaction in individuals with atopic dermatitis.

Calcineurin inhibitors: Topical medications used to reduce inflammation and itching in atopic dermatitis.

Dermatitis: Inflammation of the skin, including conditions such as atopic dermatitis.

Emollient: Moisturising agent used to hydrate and soothe the skin in atopic dermatitis.

Filaggrin: Protein important for maintaining the skin barrier function, often deficient in individuals with atopic dermatitis.

Immunoglobulin E (IgE): Antibody associated with allergic reactions, elevated in individuals with atopic dermatitis.

Keratosis pilaris: Common skin condition characterised by rough, raised bumps on the skin's surface, sometimes coexisting with atopic dermatitis.

Lichenification: Thickening and hardening of the skin in response to chronic scratching, common in atopic dermatitis.

Patch test: Diagnostic test used to identify specific allergens that may trigger atopic dermatitis flare-ups.

Phototherapy: Treatment for atopic dermatitis involving exposure to ultraviolet light to reduce inflammation and itching.

Pruritus (itch): A common symptom of atopic dermatitis characterised by the urge to scratch the skin.

Topical corticosteroids: Medications used to reduce inflammation and itching in atopic dermatitis.

Triggers: Factors or substances that can exacerbate symptoms of atopic dermatitis, such as allergens, irritants and stress.

MULTIPLE CHOICE QUESTIONS

1. Which of the following is a common symptom of atopic dermatitis?
    a) Fever
    b) Joint pain
    c) Itching
    d) Chest pain

2. What is the primary goal of skincare practices for individuals with atopic dermatitis?
    a) Enhancing skin pigmentation
    b) Reducing skin moisture
    c) Preventing sunburn
    d) Restoring the skin barrier

3. Which protein is often deficient in individuals with atopic dermatitis, leading to impaired skin barrier function?
    a) Collagen
    b) Elastin
    c) Filaggrin
    d) Keratin

4. What is the cornerstone of treatment for atopic dermatitis?
    a) Antibiotics
    b) Topical corticosteroids
    c) Moisturisers (emollients)
    d) Antihistamines

5. Which of the following is a common trigger for atopic dermatitis flare-ups?
    a) Drinking plenty of water
    b) Wearing loose-fitting clothing
    c) Exposure to stress
    d) Avoiding scratching

6. Which type of medication is commonly used to reduce inflammation and itching in atopic dermatitis?
    a) Antidepressants
    b) Antifungals
    c) Topical corticosteroids
    d) Antihypertensives

7. What is the term for the thickening and hardening of the skin in response to chronic scratching?
    a) Exfoliation
    b) Lichenification
    c) Desquamation
    d) Erosion

8. What is the primary symptom of atopic dermatitis in infants?
    a) Scaling
    b) Blistering
    c) Redness
    d) Itching

9. What role do emollients play in the management of atopic dermatitis?
    a) Reducing inflammation
    b) Preventing infection
    c) Hydrating the skin
    d) Relieving pain

10. Which environmental factor may trigger atopic dermatitis flare-ups?
   a) Exposure to sunlight
   b) Cold weather
   c) Humidity
   d) Fresh air

REFERENCES

American Academy of Dermatology Association (2023). Eczema types: atopic dermatitis causes. https://www.aad.org/public/diseases/eczema/types/atopic-dermatitis/causes (accessed May 2024).

de Lusignan, S., Alexander, H., Broderick, C. et al. (2020). The epidemiology of eczema in children and adults in England: a population-based study using primary care data. *Clinical and Experimental Allergy* 51 (3): 471–482. doi: 10.1111/cea.13784.

European Dermatology Forum (2022). Euroguiderm guideline on atopic eczema. https://www.guidelines.edf.one/uploads/attachments/clocndj4b0zskdtjrm4l247lg-atopic-eczema-gl-master-oct-2023.pdf (accessed May 2024).

Hadi, H.A., Tarmizi, A.I., Khalid, K.A. et al. (2021). The epidemiology and global burden of atopic dermatitis: a narrative review. *Life* 11 (9): 936. doi: 10.3390/life11090936.

Hale, G., Davies, E., Grindlay, D.J.C. et al. (2019). What's new in atopic eczema? An analysis of systematic reviews published in 2017. Part 2: epidemiology, aetiology and risk factors. *Clinical and Experimental Dermatology* 44 (8): 868–873. doi: 10.1111/ced.14075.

International League of Dermatological Societies (2022). Global report on atopic dermatitis 2022. https://www.eczemacouncil.org/assets/docs/global-report-on-atopic-dermatitis-2022.pdf (accessed May 2024).

Kim, J., Kim, B.E., and Leung, D.Y.M. (2019). Pathophysiology of atopic dermatitis: clinical implications. *Allergy and Asthma Proceeding* 40 (2): 84–92. doi: 10.2500/aap.2019.40.4202.

Medicines and Healthcare Products Regulatory Agency (2021). Safe use of emollient skin creams to treat dry skin conditions. https://www.gov.uk/guidance/safe-use-of-emollient-skin-creams-to-treat-dry-skin-conditions (accessed May 2021).

National Institute for Health and Care Excellence (2007). Atopic eczema in under 12s: diagnosis and management. https://www.nice.org.uk/guidance/cg57 (accessed May 2024).

Peters, J. (2019). Nursing patients with skin disorders (Chapter 13). In: *Alexander's Nursing and Practice*, 5e (ed. I. Peate). London: Elsevier.

Stephens, M. (2022). The person with a skin disorder (Chapter 35). In: *Nursing Practice*, 3e (ed. I. Peate and A. Mitchell). Oxford: Wiley.

Teasdale, E., Muller, I., Sivyer, K. et al. (2021). Views and experiences of managing eczema: systematic review and thematic synthesis of qualitative studies. *British Journal of Dermatology* 184 (4): 587–588. doi: 10.1111/bjd.19299.

Yang, L., Fu, J., and Zhou, Y. (2020). Research progress in atopic march. *Frontiers in Immunology* 11: 1907. doi:10.3389/fimmu.2020.01907.

Cancerous growth of melanocytes results in melanoma, also known as cutaneous melanoma (Scottish Intercollegiate Guidelines Network [SIGN] 2023). Melanoma is a skin cancer that arises from a skin cell called a melanocyte, which makes the pigment (melanin) that gives skin its colour. It can arise in the skin, in mucous membranes, eyes or central nervous system. Melanoma can appear in different ways, most commonly as a new spot on the skin or as an already existing mole that changes in colour, size or shape. While considered the most dangerous type of skin cancer because of its ability to spread throughout the body rapidly, melanoma is generally very treatable if it is found early (D'Orazio et al. 2013; SIGN 2023).

SKIN CANCER

Skin cancer is a broad term that encompasses cancers that develop in the skin. Cancer Research UK (CRUK 2022) notes that there are two main types of skin cancer: non-melanoma skin cancer and melanoma skin cancer. This chapter focuses on melanoma.

NON-MELANOMA SKIN CANCER

Non-melanoma skin cancer refers to all types of skin cancer that are not melanoma. The two main types of non-melanoma skin cancer are basal cell carcinoma (BCC) and squamous cell carcinoma (SCC). BCC is the most common type of skin cancer and usually appears as a flesh-coloured, pearl-like bump or a pinkish patch of skin. SCC is the second most common type and typically presents as a firm, red nodule or a flat lesion with a scaly or crusty surface. Non-melanoma skin cancers tend to develop most often on skin that has been exposed to the sun. There is a high cure rate for these cancers. Most people only have minor surgery and do not need further treatment.

MELANOMA

Melanoma can occur anywhere on the skin. Melanoma is less common than non-melanoma skin cancer but tends to be more aggressive and can spread if not treated early.

The four common subtypes are:

1. Superficial spreading melanoma (60–70%)

2. Nodular melanoma (15–30%)

3. Lentigo maligna melanoma (5–15%)

4. Acral lentiginous melanoma (5–10%)

(Cancer Research UK 2020a)

The less common forms of skin cancer include:

- Paget disease of the breast or extramammary

- Paget disease (usually in the groin or near the anus)

- Kaposi sarcoma

- Merkel cell carcinoma

- Cutaneous T-cell lymphoma

Skin cancer is the most common type of cancer (American Cancer Society 2023) and commonly develops in sun-exposed areas of skin. They can be found on any location of the body but are most commonly diagnosed on the head and neck, the areas of chronic sun exposure. The incidence is highest among people who spend a lot of time outdoors for work or recreation and is inversely related to the amount of melanin skin pigmentation; those people who have light skin are most susceptible.

MELANOCYTES

Melanocytes, located in the basal layer of the epidermis (stratum basale), extend branches between the keratinocytes in the layers above. They constitute around 5–10% of epidermal cells (see Chapter 1 of this book). While their presence is equal in both black and white skin, melanocytes in black skin produce more melanin. Variations in skin colour arise from differences in melanin quantity and the size of melanin granules produced by each melanocyte. Individuals with darker skin tones, such as dark brown or black, are less susceptible to ultraviolet (UV) radiation damage compared to those with lighter skin tones. Non-cancerous proliferation of melanocytes leads to the formation of moles (benign melanocytic naevi) and freckles (ephelides and lentigines). In contrast, the cancerous growth of melanocytes results in melanoma. Melanoma is described as:

- In situ, if a tumour remains confined to the epidermis.

- Invasive, if a tumour has extended (spread) into the dermis.

- Metastatic, indicates a tumour has spread to other tissues (DermNet NZ 2022).

Melanin serves as a protective barrier against harmful UV radiation from the sun (see Figure 5.1). Moles, clusters of melanocytes presenting as pigmented spots on the skin, can be flat or raised and round or oval. Moles (melanocytic naevi) are very common and most people have around 20–50 moles. They vary in size, shape and colour. Malignant change is uncommon; even in higher-risk groups, such as men older than 60 years of age, fewer than 1 in 33 000 moles are estimated to become malignant (Walter et al. 2010).

Although typically benign and stable, they can potentially develop into cancerous lesions. Melanoma, often indicated by changes in the size, shape or colour of an existing mole or the appearance of new moles in adulthood, requires prompt medical attention.

Not all skin offers equal sun protection, so understanding different skin types is important when offering care and support to people. An individual's vulnerability to sun-induced harm can be assessed by classifying their skin type according to the Fitzpatrick scale (Tidman and Tidman 2023) (see Table 5.1).

The Fitzpatrick scale provides a useful framework for categorising skin types based on sun sensitivity and pigmentation; it has limitations in capturing the full range of factors that contribute to an individual's susceptibility to sun-induced damage. A comprehensive assessment should consider additional factors such as environmental, behavioural and medical history to better inform sun protection recommendations and minimise the risk of skin damage. Despite its limitations, the Fitzpatrick scale remains a valuable tool to tailor sun

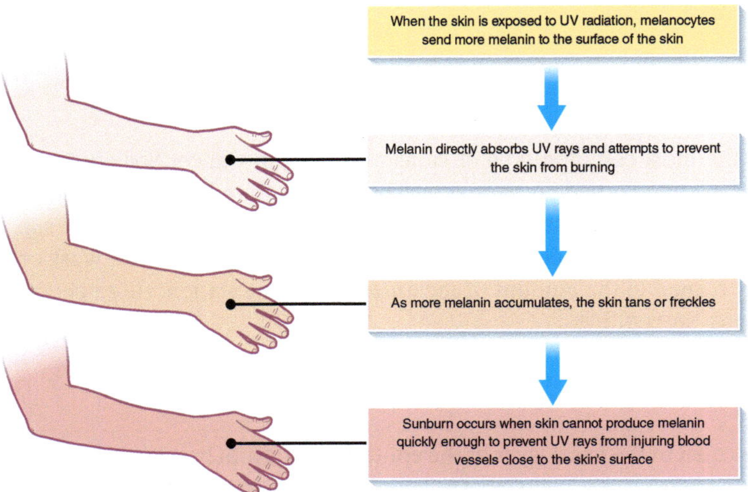

FIGURE 5.1 Melanocytes and exposure to ultraviolet radiation

Table 5.1 The Fitzpatrick scale of skin types

Type	Discussion
Type 1 (I)	Individuals with very fair skin that always burns and never tans. They typically have light-coloured eyes and hair.
Type 2 (II)	People with fair skin that burns easily and tans minimally. They often have light-coloured eyes and hair.
Type 3 (III)	Sometimes burns, usually tans. Individuals with moderately fair skin that sometimes burns and gradually tans to a light brown colour. They may have a mix of eye and hair colours. They often have light-coloured eyes and hair.
Type 4 (IV)	Always tans, occasionally burns. People with moderate brown skin that rarely burns and tans easily to a moderate brown colour. They usually have dark eyes and hair.
Type 5 (V)	Tans easily, rarely burns. Individuals with dark brown skin that rarely burns and tans very easily to a deep brown colour. They typically have dark eyes and hair.
Type 6 (VI)	Never burns, permanent deep pigmentation. Individuals with dark brown skin that rarely burns and tans very easily to a deep brown colour. They typically have dark eyes and hair.

Source: Adapted from Fitzpatrick (1988); Tidman and Tidman (2023).

protection recommendations, treatment plans for skin conditions and cosmetic procedures according to an individual's skin type.

PATHOPHYSIOLOGICAL CHANGES ASSOCIATED WITH MELANOMA

Melanoma can lead to various pathophysiological changes as it progresses. Understanding the pathophysiological changes associated with melanoma is important for early detection, accurate diagnosis, treatment selection, prognosis, development of novel therapies and long-term care and management of patients. This knowledge not only improves clinical outcomes but can also enhance the quality of care provided to individuals affected by melanoma. The pathogenesis of melanoma is complex (McCann and Huether 2019).

Melanoma is associated with a significant number of genetic mutations, a phenomenon that is known as a high mutational burden. These mutations affect genes involved in critical cellular processes such as cell cycle regulation, DNA repair and signalling pathways. The accumulation of mutations contributes to the uncontrolled growth and survival of melanoma cells.

One of the most common genetic alterations in melanoma involves the *BRAF* gene (v-Raf murine sarcoma viral oncogene homologue B), a common gene (McCann and Huether 2019). This mutation makes a pathway in cells called the MAPK (mitogen-activated protein kinase) pathway stay turned on all the time. Normally, this pathway helps control how cells grow and survive. But when it is always on, it makes melanoma cells grow too much, leading to tumour growth and spread. Besides *BRAF*, other genes can also have mutations that cause melanoma. These mutations can happen alone or together with BRAF mutations, making tumours grow and spread more.

The tumour microenvironment plays a critical role in melanoma progression and therapy resistance. It comprises various cell types, including immune cells, fibroblasts, endothelial cells and extracellular matrix components. Chronic inflammation, often driven by UV radiation, can promote tumour growth and invasion by creating a pro-tumorigenic microenvironment. While immune cells initially attempt to recognise and eliminate melanoma cells, the tumour can counteract this immune response by releasing substances that suppress immune activity. Understanding these interactions is critical for developing strategies to enhance the body's immune response against melanoma and improve treatment outcomes.

Melanoma is known for its ability to metastasise to distant organs, particularly the lungs, liver, brain and bones. Metastasis is a complex process involving several steps (see McCann and Huether 2019):

- Local invasion: Melanoma cells invade and penetrate surrounding tissues, breaking through normal tissue boundaries.

- Intravasation: Some melanoma cells enter nearby blood vessels (intravasation) or lymphatic vessels, gaining access to the circulatory or lymphatic system.

- Circulation: Once inside blood vessels or lymphatic vessels, melanoma cells travel through the bloodstream or lymphatic system to distant sites in the body.

- Extravasation: At the site of distant organs, melanoma cells exit the blood vessels or lymphatic vessels (extravasation) and enter the surrounding tissue.

- Colonisation: Finally, melanoma cells establish new tumours (metastases) in these secondary organs, where they continue to grow and proliferate.

Understanding the mechanisms underlying metastasis is essential for developing targeted therapies to prevent or treat advanced disease.

Melanoma has a propensity to provoke an immune response in the body, sometimes resulting in the spontaneous shrinking or disappearance of tumours. However, melanoma cells can develop ways to avoid detection and destruction by the immune system.

EPIDEMIOLOGY

Australia and New Zealand consistently report the highest rates of both melanoma incidence and mortality worldwide (DermNet NZ 2022). Cancer Research UK provides a range of statistical data regarding melanoma skin cancer (https://www.cancerresearchuk.org/health-professional/cancer-statistics/statistics-by-cancer-type/melanoma-skin-cancer#heading-Zero).

There were approximately 16 700 new melanoma skin cancer cases in the UK every year between 2016 and 2018. This equated to 46 cases every day. Melanoma skin cancer is the fifth most common cancer in the UK, accounting for 4% of all new cancer cases. In women in the UK, melanoma skin cancer is the fifth most common cancer. There were around 8400 new cases every year between 2016 and 2018. In men, it is the sixth most common cancer. There were 2341 deaths from melanoma skin cancer in the UK between 2017 and 2019. In England, 87% of people (2013–2017) survived melanoma skin cancer for 10 or more years.

Incidence rates for melanoma skin cancer are highest in those people aged 85–89 years. Between 2018 and 2019, more than a quarter (29%) of all new melanoma skin cancer cases were diagnosed in people aged 75 years and over.

Melanoma skin cancer incidence rates have more than doubled (140%) in the UK since the early 1990s. Rates in women have doubled (106%) and in men, they have almost tripled (186%). In the UK, in women, the most common specific location for melanoma skin cancers is the lower limb and in men, the most common specific location for melanoma skin cancers is the trunk.

Melanoma skin cancer incidence rates are projected to rise by 9% in the UK between 2023–2025 and 2038–2040. There are around 4000 cases of melanoma skin cancer each year in England that are linked with lower deprivation (around 2000 in women and around 2000 in men).

In England, incidence rates for melanoma skin cancer are lower in the Asian and Black ethnic groups, compared with the White ethnic group.

RISK FACTORS

The risk of developing melanoma depends on many things. This includes lifestyle factors and some medical conditions. Melanoma risk factors can be broadly categorised into environmental, genetic and personal factors (CRUK 2020b; Hagler et al. 2023; SIGN 2023).

ULTRAVIOLET RADIATION EXPOSURE

Exposure to UV radiation from the sun or artificial sources (such as tanning beds) is one of the most significant risk factors for melanoma. Intense, intermittent sun exposure, particularly leading to sunburn during childhood or adolescence, is associated with an increased risk.

FAIR SKIN, HAIR AND EYES

Individuals with fair skin, light hair (blonde or red) and light-coloured eyes (blue or green) have less natural protection against UV radiation and are at higher risk of developing melanoma (those with Fitzpatrick skin type I and II; see Table 5.1) compared to those with darker skin tones. People with black or brown skin can still get melanoma; however, they have more natural protection against it. Melanoma is uncommon among individuals with black or brown skin in the UK. However, if it does occur, it typically manifests as acral lentiginous melanoma, which commonly develops on the soles of the feet or palms of the hands. It can also appear under the nail.

PERSONAL OR FAMILY HISTORY

A personal history of melanoma or other skin cancers increases the risk of developing melanoma. Additionally, having a first-degree relative (parent, sibling or child) with a history of melanoma also elevates an individual's risk.

PRESENCE OF ATYPICAL MOLES (DYSPLASTIC NAEVI)

Atypical moles are unusual-looking moles that may exhibit irregular borders, asymmetry, variegated colour and larger size compared to common moles. Having a higher number of atypical moles increases the risk of melanoma. Although the presence of numerous moles increases the risk of melanoma, the majority of melanomas do not originate from existing moles but instead arise as new growths on the skin.

WEAKENED IMMUNE SYSTEM

Individuals with weakened immune systems, such as those undergoing immunosuppressive therapy following organ transplantation or individuals with conditions such as human immunodeficiency virus, have an increased risk of developing melanoma.

PREVIOUS RADIATION THERAPY

Previous exposure to radiation therapy for the treatment of other cancers may increase the risk of developing melanoma in the irradiated area.

CERTAIN GENETIC FACTORS

Specific genetic mutations, such as mutations in the *BRAF* genes, can predispose individuals to melanoma. Additionally, inherited conditions such as familial atypical multiple mole melanoma syndrome and xeroderma pigmentosum are associated with an increased risk of melanoma.

AGE AND GENDER

Melanoma can occur at any age but is more commonly diagnosed in older individuals. Additionally, men have a higher overall risk of developing melanoma compared to women, although rates among younger individuals may be higher in women.

GEOGRAPHIC LOCATION

Living closer to the equator or at higher altitudes with increased UV radiation exposure may increase the risk of melanoma.

OCCUPATIONAL EXPOSURE

Certain occupations with outdoor work or exposure to chemicals may increase the risk of melanoma. Polychlorinated biphenyls have been identified as substances that can heighten the risk of developing melanoma skin cancer. These chemicals are present in certain outdated electrical equipment.

Understanding the risk factors can help individuals and those who offer care and support identify those at higher risk and implement appropriate prevention strategies, including sun protection measures, regular skin examinations and early detection efforts.

CLINICAL PRESENTATION

Melanomas can emerge anywhere on the body, not exclusively in regions exposed to sunlight. In the UK, the trunk is the most prevalent site for men, while the leg is the most common location for women (CRUK 2020a).

While melanoma typically commences as a skin lesion, it can also manifest on mucous membranes, such as the lips or genitals (known as mucosal melanoma). In some cases, it may arise in other areas of the body, including the eyes, brain, mouth or vagina. The initial

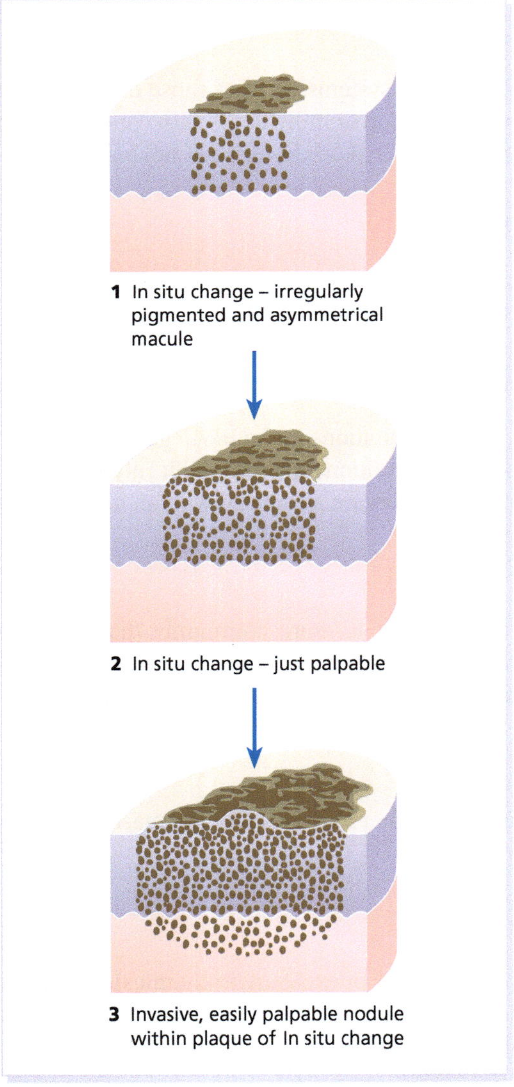

FIGURE 5.2 Radial intraepidermal growth phase of melanoma (1 and 2) precedes vertical and invasive dermal growth phase (3).

indication of melanoma typically presents as an unusual-looking freckle or mole, often accompanied by itching or bleeding. Melanomas may expand horizontally across the skin (radial growth phase; see Figure 5.2) or vertically into deeper layers (vertical growth phase). Melanoma can be detected at an early stage when it is only a few millimetres in diameter, although it may enlarge to several centimetres before diagnosis. Melanomas can exhibit various colours, including tan, dark brown, black, blue, red and occasionally light grey. Some melanomas lack pigment and are termed amelanotic melanomas. Additionally, there may be areas of regression that resemble normal skin colour or appear white and scarred (DermNet NZ 2022).

During the horizontal growth phase, melanomas typically appear flat. As the vertical growth phase progresses, they become thickened, raised and palpable. Some melanomas may cause itching or tenderness, while more advanced lesions may bleed easily or form crusts.

ABCDE EFG AND 7-POINT CHECK LIST

Most melanomas have characteristics that can be described by using the ABCDE EFG melanoma criteria or the 7-point checklist.

THE ABCDE EFG OF MELANOMA

For superficial melanomas, the ABCDE EFG mnemonic is a tool used to help recognise potential signs of melanoma. Each letter corresponds to a specific characteristic that may indicate the presence of melanoma (DermNet NZ 2022):

A: Asymmetry of shape and colour. One half of the lesion does not match the other half in shape or size.

B: Border irregularity. Including smudgy, jagged or ill-defined margin.

C: Colour variation and change. The mole exhibits multiple colours or shades, such as brown, black, blue, red or white.

D: Different/diameter. The diameter is larger than approximately 6 mm or more.

E: Evolving (enlarging). There has been a change in size, shape, colour or elevation over time.

Melanomas may not conform to the 'ABCDE' rule alone. Not all melanomas exhibit these specific characteristics. In other words, there may be melanomas that do not fit neatly into the ABCDE criteria but are still concerning for skin cancer. This highlights the importance of being vigilant for any suspicious skin lesions, even if they do not perfectly match the ABCD criteria.

For nodular melanomas (which often present as raised or elevated lesions with a firm texture and rapid growth), the EFG signs should also be considered (DermNet NZ 2022):

E: Elevated. Raised or elevated from the skin surface.

F: Firm to touch. Feels firm or hard when touched.

G: Growing. Progressively increasing in size over time.

Taking a thorough history is important, and any lesion that changes in size, shape, colour or elevation for more than one month should be reviewed by a dermatologist or biopsied.

Table 5.2 The 7-point checklist

Major features (two points each)	Minor features (one point each)
• Change in size of lesion	• Inflammation
• Irregular pigmentation	• Itch/altered sensation
• Irregular border	• Lesion larger than others
	• Oozing/crusting of lesion

Source: Adapted from SIGN (2023).

7-POINT CHECKLIST

Distinguishing malignant from benign pigmented skin lesions in practice can be challenging. The weighted 7-point checklist is a single-site cancer decision support tool that can be used in assessing patients (often those in primary care) who present with pigmented skin lesions. Suspicious pigmented lesions should be assessed using the 7-point checklist (see Table 5.2).

Any patient with a score of 3 or more on the 7-point checklist, a suspected cancer pathway referral should be considered (National Institute for Health and Care Excellence 2023).

CLINICAL INVESTIGATIONS AND DIAGNOSIS

Peters (2019) notes that early detection and excision of thin tumours (less than 1 mm thick) carry an excellent prognosis and potential cure. Untreated melanoma that has advanced to late stages with metastases typically results in a less favourable prognosis and treatment primarily focuses on palliative care, such as radiotherapy.

The diagnosis of melanoma involves history taking, physical examination and there may be a need for further clinical investigations to be undertaken to accurately assess suspicious skin lesions.

HISTORY TAKING

History taking is a key component of the diagnostic process for melanoma. During the patient interview, information is gathered about the patient's medical history, personal habits and potential risk factors for melanoma.

There is no national screening programme for melanoma skin cancer in the UK. This is because research has not yet determined if the benefits of screening outweigh the risks. The most effective way to detect melanoma early is for individuals to be aware of the symptoms and consult a healthcare professional (for example, a practice nurse or general practitioner [GP]) if they notice any concerning signs (CRUK 2024).

Any previous diagnoses of skin cancer, including melanoma, as well as other medical conditions that may increase the risk of melanoma, such as immunosuppression or genetic syndromes associated with melanoma predisposition (e.g. familial atypical multiple mole melanoma syndrome) are discussed.

Inquiring about a family history of melanoma or other skin cancers is important, as individuals with first-degree relatives (parents, siblings or children) who have had melanoma are at higher risk of developing the condition themselves. A positive family history may prompt more frequent surveillance and earlier intervention for suspicious lesions.

The patient is asked about sun exposure habits, including occupational exposure, recreational sun exposure and history of sunburn. This can help to assess the cumulative UV radiation exposure, which is a major risk factor for melanoma. Intermittent, intense sun exposure leading to sunburn, especially during childhood or adolescence, increases the risk of developing melanoma later in life.

Indoor tanning (use of tanning beds) is associated with an increased risk of melanoma and other skin cancers, particularly when initiated at a young age. Inquiries about indoor tanning practices and sun protection behaviours, such as sunscreen use, protective clothing and seeking shade, provide insights into modifiable risk factors for melanoma.

Patients may report changes in the size, colour, shape or texture of existing moles or the appearance of new lesions on the skin. Asking about the evolution of these changes over time helps assess the likelihood of melanoma and guides further clinical evaluation and management.

Those patients with advanced melanoma may experience symptoms such as itching, tenderness, pain or bleeding at the site of a skin lesion. Inquiring about these symptoms helps identify lesions that may require closer examination or biopsy.

Gathering information through history taking can help with further assessment (the physical examination) of the patient as well as their risk profile, identify potential signs and symptoms of melanoma and tailor the diagnostic approach accordingly. A comprehensive history provides valuable context for clinical evaluation, dermoscopy and biopsy, ultimately contributing to the early detection and diagnosis of melanoma.

PHYSICAL EXAMINATION

During the consultation, the patient's skin will be carefully examined. DermNet NZ (2022) notes that melanoma may be suspected because of a lesion's clinical features or a history of change.

It is essential that issues relating to consent, the provision of a chaperone, maintaining dignity and comfort and adherence to infection prevention and control policies and procedures are all adhered to. During the physical examination, the following may be performed:

- The mole or abnormal area of skin is measured with a ruler or against a marker scale.

- A photograph may be taken, so any changes can be recorded.

- A dermoscope is used to examine the mole or abnormal area of skin. This is an instrument that contains a light and magnifying lens to better visualise skin spots.

- The mole or abnormal area of skin is compared to other moles or other areas of the patient's skin.

CLINICAL INVESTIGATIONS

A skin biopsy will be undertaken if there is a suspicion of melanoma, other types of skin cancer or any skin abnormalities. During this procedure, a sample of the suspicious area is removed for microscopic examination to check for cancer cells. Occasionally, to confirm a melanoma diagnosis or to further analyse the genetic characteristics of melanoma cells (which can influence treatment and prognosis), additional tests on the biopsy sample may be performed in the laboratory.

Lymph node ultrasound and biopsy uses high-frequency sound waves to examine lymph nodes. This investigation may be performed to determine if melanoma skin cancer has spread from the skin to the lymph nodes. A sample biopsy may be taken from the lymph node if it looks abnormal.

If a sentinel lymph node biopsy is required, it is performed at the same time as the surgical procedure to remove the skin and tissue around the site of the melanoma. This operation is called a wide local excision. Sentinel lymph node biopsy (these are the first lymph node or nodes that a cancer may spread to) for melanoma skin cancer is a test to identify these lymph nodes (CRUK 2020a).

Table 5.3 discusses other interventions that may be used to support a diagnosis.

The diagnosis of melanoma requires a comprehensive approach involving clinical examination, dermoscopy, biopsy and histopathological examination. Early detection and accurate diagnosis are crucial for timely intervention and optimal management of melanoma.

Table 5.3   Supporting interventions that may be used to make diagnosis of melanoma

Intervention	Discussion
Dermoscopy	Identifying certain melanomas clinically can be challenging. Dermoscopic evaluation aids in their diagnosis. Specific criteria for melanoma often encompass an abnormal pigment network, brown–black dots/globules, multiple (five to six) colours that are unevenly spread, a blue–white veil, depigmentation and an irregular vascular pattern. Dermoscopic monitoring is appropriate for flat or slightly elevated lesions, while any suspicious or nodular lesions warrant excision.
Confocal microscopy	Confocal microscopy is an advanced imaging technique used in dermatology for non-invasive examination of skin lesions at a cellular level. Unlike traditional microscopy, which captures images of multiple layers of tissue simultaneously, confocal microscopy selectively focuses on a specific plane within the skin, allowing for high-resolution imaging of individual cells and structures._ Where available, confocal microscopy may be useful for clinical and dermoscopic examination of suspected melanoma lesions. Confocal microscopy offers valuable insights into skin pathology. Its widespread use in clinical practice is limited by factors such as equipment cost, operator expertise and the need for validation studies to establish diagnostic accuracy and reliability.
Photographic skin surveillance	Where this is available, total body photography, such as MoleMap, should be considered for high-risk individuals, especially those with numerous naevi and dysplastic naevi. Total body photography establishes a baseline for tracking new lesions and changes in existing ones.
Radiographic investigations	Imaging techniques, for example, CT or PET scans, may be suitable for staging or monitoring melanomas that carry a high risk of distant metastasis.
Adhesive patch genomic analysis	Skin surface tape stripping is a non-invasive test that can be used on pigmented lesions to obtain their genomic signature, aiding in the diagnosis of melanoma.

Source: Adapted from DermNet NZ (2022).

STAGING

The stage of melanoma describes how thick (deep) it is and if it has spread from where it started. The way melanoma is staged is complicated, for example:

- The number of stages from 0 to 4 (see Table 5.4)

- Breslow thickness (see Table 5.5)

- Tumour, nodes, metastasises (TNM) staging (see Table 5.6)

After a melanoma diagnosis, the next step taken is to stage the cancer. Staging is a critical process as it determines how deeply the melanoma has penetrated the skin and the extent to which it has spread to other parts of the body. This information is essential for developing an effective treatment plan. Melanoma is categorised into the stages identified in Table 5.4.

National Institute for Health and Care Excellence (2023) has recommended that a person should receive a diagnosis or ruling out of cancer within 28 days of being referred urgently by their GP for suspected cancer. Each stage of melanoma requires a tailored approach to treatment, which may include surgery, immunotherapy, targeted therapy, radiation therapy or a combination of these. Early detection and accurate staging are crucial for improving the prognosis and survival rates of individuals diagnosed with melanoma.

Table 5.4 Staging of melanoma

Stage	Discussion
Stage 0 (melanoma in situ)	At this earliest stage, melanoma is confined to the outermost layer of the skin (epidermis) and has not yet invaded deeper layers.
Stage 1	In this stage, melanoma has begun to invade the dermis but is still relatively small and thin, typically less than 2 mm thick. It may or may not be ulcerated.
Stage 2	Here, melanoma is thicker and may range from 2 to 4 mm or more. It can be ulcerated or non-ulcerated, indicating a higher risk of spreading.
Stage 3	Melanoma at this stage has spread to nearby lymph nodes or tissues around the original tumour site but has not yet reached distant organs. The tumour may be any thickness and might be ulcerated.
Stage 4	This advanced stage means melanoma has spread to distant lymph nodes or other organs such as the lungs, liver, brain or distant parts of the skin. It represents the most serious form of melanoma.

Source: Adapted from MacMillan (2022).

Table 5.5 Breslow thickness

Levels of tumour thickness	Discussion
Tis	The melanoma cells are only in the very top layer of the skin (epidermis).
T1	The melanoma is 1 mm thick or less.
T2	The melanoma is between 1 and 2 mm thick.
T3	The melanoma is between 2 and 4 mm thick.
T4	The melanoma is more than 4 mm thick.

Source: Adapted from MacMillan (2022).

Table 5.6 TNM staging for melanoma

Stage	Discussion
T (tumour)	Describes the thickness of the melanoma. This is also called the Breslow thickness.
N (node)	N stands for nodes and nearby skin. It describes if the melanoma has spread to nearby lymph nodes. It also describes any spread to areas of skin between the tumour and these lymph nodes. This is called in-transit, satellite or microsatellite metastases.
	• N0: the melanoma has not spread from where it started.
	• N1: the melanoma has spread to one lymph node or to nearby areas of skin.
	• N2: the melanoma has spread to two or three lymph nodes or to one lymph node and nearby skin.
	• N3: the melanoma has spread to four or more lymph nodes or to two or more lymph nodes and nearby skin or to any number of lymph nodes and these have stuck together.
M (metastasis)	M stands for metastases and describes whether the melanoma has spread to other parts of the body, for example, the lungs, liver, bones, brain or distant areas of the skin. This is also known as advanced or metastatic cancer.
	• M0: the melanoma has not spread to other parts of the body.
	• M1: the melanoma has spread to other parts of the body.

Source: Adapted from MacMillan (2022).

MANAGEMENT

Treatment options are decided upon with the patient at the centre of all that is done. A multi-disciplinary approach is adopted, involving specialist nurses, oncologists and dermatologists in providing care. Treatment depends primarily on how deeply the melanoma has grown, whether the cancer has spread, where the cancer is located and the patient's overall health (CRUK 2020c). Most patients will undergo surgery to remove additional tissue from the area where the mole was excised. If detected early, 90% of melanomas can be cured with this straightforward surgical procedure (DermNet NZ 2022). This surgery, wide local excision, aims to remove all cancer cells. For early-stage melanoma (stages 0, 1 and 2), this is often the only treatment required. Early-stage melanoma indicates that the cancer cells are confined to the skin and have not spread beyond the original site of the mole (MacMillan 2022).

The surgical procedure undertaken may also include a biopsy of a nearby lymph node to evaluate whether the melanoma has spread. If melanoma has spread to nearby lymph nodes, regular ultrasounds of the lymph nodes may be the best option. These ultrasounds check if the cancer is growing in that area and if further treatment is needed. More advanced melanomas (these are stage 3 or 4) may necessitate a combination of treatments, including surgery, drug therapy and radiation therapy. All patients with melanoma with distant metastases are evaluated by a multidisciplinary team to determine the best treatment plan.

Table 5.7 outlines the treatment options by stage. To reiterate, treatment is decided upon with the patient and based on the person's individual needs.

After treatment, follow-up appointments are needed depending on the stage of the melanoma. There may be a one-off follow-up appointment, for example, with stage 0 melanoma. For other stages of melanoma, regular appointments over several years may be required.

Table 5.7 Treatment options

Stage	Treatment options
Stage 0 (melanoma in situ)	Surgery is the main treatment. Melanoma is diagnosed by biopsy. A second procedure may be needed to remove a larger area of healthy tissue around where the melanoma was (a wide local excision). This is all the treatment needed. Regular ultrasound scans of the lymph nodes to check if the cancer has progressed (known as surveillance). Ultrasound surveillance is usually for five years.
Stages 1 and 2	Stages 1 and 2 are early cancers in the skin and have not spread to other parts of the body. Surgery is the main treatment, wide local excision. Lymph node staging and sentinel lymph node biopsy may be performed, usually under a general anaesthetic. If melanoma is found, removal of the lymph node(s) may be considered.
Stage 3	Stage 3 melanoma skin cancer indicates that the cancer cells have spread to the nearby lymph nodes or to the tissue between the melanoma and these lymph nodes. After being diagnosed with melanoma, a wide local excision is performed to remove more tissue in the area where the melanoma was. When melanoma spreads from the primary tumour to nearby lymph nodes, the spread is termed satellite or in-transit metastases, based on their distance from the original melanoma. Surgery is the primary treatment. If the patient is unable to undergo surgery, one of the following may be considered: • Laser surgery using a carbon dioxide laser • Injecting directly into the melanoma (intralesional therapy), for example talimogene laherparepvec (T-VEC) • Chemotherapy that is combined with an electric current (electrochemotherapy) • Chemotherapy directly into the leg or arm where the melanoma is (known as isolated limb infusion or isolated limb perfusion) • Targeted cancer drugs • Immunotherapy • Chemotherapy If melanoma cells are detected in the nearby lymph nodes by sentinel lymph node biopsy, the following may be considered: • Regular ultrasound scans • Targeted cancer drugs or immunotherapy If there are swollen or abnormal looking lymph nodes and a biopsy has confirmed the melanoma has spread to the lymph nodes, then lymph node dissection or lymphadenectomy can be performed. Treatment after surgery can be offered, which is known as adjuvant treatment. This may be required for up to one year. The aim is to reduce the risk of the cancer coming back.

(Continued)

Table 5.7 (*Continued*)

Stage	Treatment options
Stage 4	In stage 4, the cancer has spread to other parts of the body, such as the liver, which is also called advanced melanoma. The patient may be offered one or more of the following treatments to help control the cancer and its symptoms: • Surgery • Targeted cancer drugs • Immunotherapy • Radiotherapy to specific sites of melanoma spread, for example the bone or brain • Injection of a drug directly into the melanoma (intralesional therapy), for example, talimogene laherparepvec (T-VEC) • Chemotherapy directly into the leg or arm where the melanoma is • Chemotherapy that is combined with an electric current (electrochemotherapy) • Chemotherapy, usually the patient will only have chemotherapy if they are unable to have a targeted cancer drug or immunotherapy
Some patients may be asked to take part in clinical trials as part of their treatment.	

Source: Adapted from CRUK (2020c); MacMillan (2022).

Some patients will be offered regular scans if there is a higher risk of melanoma coming back and needing treatment.

The patient's skin is carefully examined during follow-up appointments. After a melanoma, there is a higher risk of the person getting another one. Photographs of the skin are taken and measurements of moles are recorded. This is done so as to check for any changes in the skin. The areas where melanoma was removed for signs of it coming back to the same place are also checked. The scar around the surrounding area is examined as well as the lymph nodes closest to where the melanoma was, as well as lymph nodes elsewhere in the body.

HEALTH TEACHING

Health education for people with melanoma is crucial for helping them understand their condition, manage treatment and take preventive measures to reduce the risk of recurrence. Excessive ultraviolet radiation from the sun can harm skin cells and lead to skin cancer. In the UK, nearly 9 out of 10 melanoma skin cancer cases could be prevented by practising sun safety and avoiding sunbeds (CRUK 2023). Regardless of location, protection from the sun is crucial. In the UK, the sun's rays can be strong enough to cause damage between mid-March and mid-October, even on cold or cloudy days.

Those who provide care and support should offer people information on what melanoma is, its stages and how it progresses. An explanation of prognosis based on stage and individual health factors is required.

Provide information about the role of genetic mutations (e.g. BRAF) and how they influence treatment options. Explanations of surgical options, immunotherapy, targeted therapy, chemotherapy and radiation therapy so people can make informed decisions.

Discuss strategies that may help with the management of common side effects of treatments, such as fatigue, nausea, skin reactions and immune-related side effects from immunotherapy. It is vital to emphasise the importance of adhering to treatment schedules and follow-up appointments.

Explain to patients how to perform regular self-examinations to detect new moles or changes in existing ones. Explain the signs and symptoms of recurrence or complications that require prompt medical attention. Table 5.8 discusses the components of self-examination.

Regularly performing the self-examination steps detailed in Table 5.8 can help to detect potential skin issues early, promptly seeking medical advice can improve the chances of successful treatment.

Instilling the importance of sun protection, including the use of sunscreen, protective clothing and avoiding peak sun exposure times, can help to reduce the risk of melanoma.

Table 5.8 Self-examination to detect new moles or changes in existing ones

Component	Discussion
Preparation	Lighting: ensure there is good lighting, preferably natural light or a bright overhead light.
	Mirrors: use a full-length mirror and a hand-held mirror to examine hard-to-see areas.
	Tools: have a notebook or a camera to record findings and a ruler to measure moles.
What to look for	New moles: check for any new moles or growths on the skin.
	Changes in existing moles: look for changes in size, shape, colour or texture of existing moles.
	Use ABCDE rule to evaluate moles:
	A: asymmetry
	B: border
	C: colour
	D: diameter
	E: evolving
Examination steps	Face and scalp: use a comb or blow-dryer to part the hair and check the scalp. Check the face, including ears and neck.
	Torso: examine the front and back of the body in the mirror. Lift the breasts to check the skin underneath.
	Arms: check forearms, underarms and upper arms, using a hand mirror for hard-to-see areas.
	Hands: examine palms, backs of the hands, between the fingers and under the fingernails.
	Legs: look at the front and back of the legs, as well as the backs of the thighs using a hand mirror if necessary.
	Feet: inspect the tops, soles, between the toes and under the toenails.
	Back and buttocks: use a hand mirror to check the back, buttocks and genital area.

(Continued)

Table 5.8 (*Continued*)

Component	Discussion
Recording findings	Note changes: write down any changes observed, including the date, description and measurements of moles.
	Take photos: photograph moles and areas of concern to compare over time. Ensure photographs are clear and taken from the same angle each time.
Frequency	Perform a self-examination once a month to become familiar with the skin and detect any changes early.
When to report findings	A healthcare professional (for example, dermatologist, practice nurse, GP) should be consulted: If any new, unusual or changing moles or any other skin changes are noticed, which give a cause for concern.
A partner can also help (if willing) to help perform a self-skin check.	

Source: Adapted from Murchie et al. (2015).

Encouraging a healthy diet, regular exercise and smoking cessation can help to improve overall health and potentially reduce cancer recurrence risk.

Address the emotional impact of a melanoma diagnosis and provide resources for coping strategies, support groups and counselling services. Encourage open communication with those who offer care and support about fears, concerns and questions related to melanoma. If appropriate, involve family members in information giving sessions to ensure they understand the patient's needs and can offer support.

Addressing the various healthcare needs of people with melanoma can empower patients with this condition to take an active role in their care, improving their outcomes and quality of life.

CONCLUSION

Offering care and support to individuals with melanoma requires a multifaceted approach that encompasses education, prevention, early detection, treatment and ongoing support. It is important to develop a thorough understanding of melanoma and its management. Discussion with and providing information to patients about the risk factors, signs and symptoms of melanoma, as well as promoting sun safety practices and regular skin self-examinations can empower individuals to take an active role in their health and well-being.

Promoting empathy, compassion and cultural competence in caring for patients with melanoma is essential for improving positive patient outcomes and enhancing the overall quality of care. Collaboration with interdisciplinary healthcare teams and engagement in ongoing professional development can demonstrate a commitment to delivering patient-centred care that is holistic, compassionate and evidence-based.

GLOSSARY OF TERMS

7-point checklist: A tool used to assess pigmented skin lesions for signs of melanoma.

ABCDE EFG rule: A mnemonic used to assess moles and lesions for signs of melanoma:

Asymmetry
Border irregularity
Colour variation

Diameter greater than 6 mm

Evolution or change over time

For nodular melanomas, the EFG signs should also be considered

Elevated: raised or elevated from the skin surface

Firm to touch: feels firm or hard when touched

Growing: progressively increasing in size over time

Biopsy: A procedure to remove a sample of tissue for examination under a microscope to determine if it is cancerous.

Chemotherapy: Treatment that uses drugs to kill cancer cells or stop them from growing.

Dermatologist: A medical doctor who specialises in diagnosing and treating skin disorders, including melanoma.

Immunotherapy: Treatment that uses the body's immune system to fight cancer.

Melanocytes: Cells that produce melanin, the pigment responsible for skin colour, and can become cancerous, leading to melanoma.

Metastasis: The spread of cancer from one part of the body to another, often through the lymphatic system or bloodstream.

Radiation therapy: Treatment that uses high-energy rays to kill cancer cells or stop them from growing.

Sentinel lymph node biopsy: A procedure to remove and examine the lymph node(s) most likely to contain cancer cells from a primary tumour.

Skin self-examination: Regular inspection of the skin to monitor for changes in existing moles or the development of new ones.

Sunscreen: A topical product applied to the skin to protect it from the harmful effects of ultraviolet (UV) radiation from the sun.

Surgical excision: Removal of the entire melanoma along with a margin of normal tissue to ensure complete removal of cancer cells.

Targeted therapy: Treatment that uses drugs or other substances to specifically target cancer cells while minimising damage to normal cells.

Wide local excision: Surgical removal of the melanoma along with a margin of healthy tissue to reduce the risk of recurrence.

MULTIPLE CHOICE QUESTIONS

1. What is the primary risk factor for developing melanoma?
   a) Smoking
   b) Obesity
   c) Excessive sun exposure
   d) Family history of diabetes

2. What is the recommended size threshold for monitoring moles for signs of melanoma?
   a) 2 mm
   b) 4 mm
   c) 6 mm
   d) 8 mm

3. What is the gold standard diagnostic procedure for melanoma?
   a) Blood test
   b) MRI scan
   c) Biopsy
   d) Urinalysis

4. What is the primary goal of surgery in treating melanoma?
   a) To relieve pain
   b) To remove the entire tumour
   c) To prevent infection
   d) To improve appetite

5. What is the first step in the ABCDE rule for assessing moles for signs of melanoma?
   a) Evolution
   b) Asymmetry
   c) Border irregularity
   d) Colour variation

6. What does the 'E' stand for in the ABCDE rule?
   a) Elevated
   b) Evolution
   c) Excessive bleeding
   d) Exudate

7. Which treatment modality uses high-energy rays to kill cancer cells?
   a) Immunotherapy
   b) Surgery
   c) Radiation therapy
   d) Targeted therapy

8. Which procedure involves removing and examining the lymph node(s) most likely to contain cancer cells?
   a) Sentinel lymph node biopsy
   b) Mohs surgery
   c) Wide local excision
   d) Chemotherapy

9. What is the purpose of the 7-point checklist in assessing pigmented skin lesions?
   a) To diagnose melanoma definitively
   b) To classify moles as benign or malignant
   c) To assess the risk of metastasis
   d) To identify suspicious lesions that may require further evaluation

10. What is the term for the surgical removal of the entire melanoma along with a margin of normal tissue?
    a) Chemotherapy
    b) Mohs surgery
    c) Wide local excision
    d) Radiation therapy

REFERENCES

American Cancer Society (2023). Key statistics for basal and squamous cell skin cancers. https://www.cancer.org/cancer/types/basal-and-squamous-cell-skin-cancer/about/key-statistics.html (accessed May 2024).

Cancer Research UK (2020a). Tests for melanoma skin cancer. https://www.cancerresearchuk.org/about-cancer/melanoma/getting-diagnosed/tests-stage (accessed May 2024).

Cancer Research UK (2020b). Tests to stage. https://www.cancerresearchuk.org/about-cancer/melanoma/getting-diagnosed/tests-melanoma Tests for melanoma skin cancer | Cancer Research UK (accessed December 2024).

Cancer Research UK (2020c). Treatment options. https://www.cancerresearchuk.org/about-cancer/melanoma/treatment/treatment-decisions (accessed May 2024).

Cancer Research UK (2022). Melanoma skin cancer. https://www.cancerresearchuk.org/about-cancer/melanoma (accessed May 2024).

Cancer Research UK (2023). Sun safety. https://www.cancerresearchuk.org/about-cancer/causes-of-cancer/sun-uv-and-cancer/sun-safety (accessed May 2024).

Cancer Research UK (2024). Screening for melanoma skin cancer. https://www.cancerresearchuk.org/about-cancer/melanoma/getting-diagnosed/screening (accessed May 2024).

DermNet NZ (2022). Melanoma. Melanoma skin cancer: images, diagnosis, and treatment. https://dermnetnz.org/topics/melanoma (accessed May 2024).

D'Orazio, J., Jarrett, S., Amaro-Ortiz, A. et al. (2013). UV radiation and the skin. *International Journal of Molecular Sciences* 14 (6): 12222–12248. https://www.mdpi.com/1422-0067/14/6/12222.

Fitzpatrick, T.B. (1988). The validity and practicality of sun-reactive skin types I through VI. *Archives of Dermatology* 124 (6): 869–871.

Hagler, D., Harding, M.M., Kwong, J. et al. (2023). *Lewis's Medical-Surgical Nursing*. St Louis: Elsevier.

MacMillan (2022). Staging of melanoma – TNM staging and Breslow thickness. https://www.macmillan.org.uk/cancer-information-and-support/melanoma/staging-of-melanoma (accessed May 2024).

McCann, S.A. and Huether, S.E. (2019). Structure, function, and disorders of the integument (Chapter 47). In: *Pathophysiology the Biologic Basis for Disease in Adults and Children*, 8e (ed. K.L. McCance and S.E. Huether). St Louis: Elsevier.

Murchie, P., Allan, J.L., Brant, W. et al. (2015). Total skin self-examination at home for people treated for cutaneous melanoma: development and pilot of a digital intervention. *BMJ Open* 5 (8): e007993. doi: 10.1136/bmjopen-2015-007993.

National Institute for Health and Care Excellence (2023). Suspected cancer: recognition and referral suspected cancer. https://www.nice.org.uk/guidance/ng12/resources/suspected-cancer-recognition-and-referral-pdf-1837268071621 (accessed May 2024).

Peters, J. (2019). Nursing patients with skin disorders (Chapter 13). In: *Alexanders's Nursing Practice*, 5e (ed. I. Peate). London: Elsevier.

Scottish Intercollegiate Guidelines Network (2023). Cutaneous melanoma. https://www.sign.ac.uk/media/2108/sign-146-cutaneous-melanoma-2023.pdf (accessed May 2024).

Tidman, M.J. and Tidman, A.S.M. (2023). The skin, hair and nails (Chapter 14). In: *MacLeod's Clinical Examination*, 15e (ed. A.R. Dover, A.R. Innes, and K. Fairhurst). London: Elsevier.

Walter, F.M., Humphrys, E., Tso, S. et al. (2010). Patient understanding of moles and skin cancer, and factors influencing presentation in primary care: a qualitative study. *BMC Family Practice* 11. 62. doi: 10.1186/1471-2296-11-620.

Burns are injuries to the skin or other tissues resulting from thermal, radiation, chemical or electrical exposure. A scald is a burn caused by contact with a hot liquid or steam (World Health Organization [WHO] 2023). Burns are a significant global public health issue, responsible for an estimated 180 000 deaths annually. The majority of these fatalities occur in low- and middle-income countries, with nearly two-thirds happening in the WHO African and South-East Asia Regions. In many high-income countries, burn mortality rates have been declining, but the rate of child deaths from burns is still over seven times higher in low- and middle-income countries compared to high-income countries. Non-fatal burns are a major cause of morbidity, leading to prolonged hospitalisation, disfigurement, disability and often result in stigma and social rejection. Burns are among the leading causes of disability-adjusted life years lost in low- and middle-income countries (WHO 2023).

FIRST AID FOR BURNS

Burn injuries result from the transfer of energy from a heat source to vulnerable tissues. The higher the temperature of the heat source is and the longer that it remains in contact with the tissues, the more severe the damage will be. The prompt and effective application of first aid for burns can positively influence burn outcomes by preventing further tissue damage and reducing subsequent morbidity.

The first priority in first aid treatment is to remove the person from the heat source. If the cause is electricity, then turn off the power supply if possible or use a non-conductive material to rescue the person. Often, there is a continuing heat source if the person's clothing is on fire or soaked with hot liquid. The most effective way to eliminate this ongoing heat source is to douse the affected area with a cool liquid that is neither flammable nor corrosive, extinguishing the flames or lowering the temperature of the hot liquid. If such a liquid is not available, quickly removing the hot, soaked clothing will stop the heat transfer. If clothing is on fire, prevent the person from running around, which can fan the flames. Lay the person on the ground and use a heavy material, such as a coat or blanket, to smother the flames (McCahill 2019).

If chemicals are the cause, promptly rinse with large amounts of water to dilute the chemical and limit its penetration into the skin, where it can cause prolonged damage, taking care not to wash chemicals into the eyes (McCann, Watson, and Barnes 2022). Chemicals such as hydrofluoric acid, which are frequently used in both industrial and domestic environments, require treatment with specific neutralising agents when they cause injuries. Hydrofluoric acid is particularly dangerous and can penetrate skin, causing severe damage. Therefore, its treatment often involves the use of specific substances designed to neutralise the acid and mitigate its harmful effects, rather than application of general first aid measures such as rinsing with water (Huang et al. 2021).

After removing the heat source, the next step is to cool the superheated tissues. The British Burn Association (2018) advises applying cool running tap water to the affected area for 20 minutes. Cooling is beneficial for up to three hours after the injury and should still be performed even if there is a delay in accessing cooling methods. For the face, use cold soaks instead. Wright, Harris, and Furniss (2015) suggest avoiding the use of ice or water below 8 °C, as this increases the likelihood of tissue damage. Continued cooling helps reduce pain from the burn wound, but if a large body area is involved, there is a risk of hypothermia. Those patients with extensive burns have difficulty retaining body heat, so using space blankets or other heat-retaining coverings is recommended during transfer to the hospital.

Many burn associations suggest using polyvinyl chloride film (e.g. cling film) as a temporary wound cover while awaiting transfer to the emergency department or a dedicated burn service (McLure et al. 2021). Polyvinyl chloride film:

- Does not stick to the wound and cause pain upon removal.

- Conforms closely to body contours and excludes air, reducing pain.

- Allows the wound to be viewed without removing the film.

However, cling film should only be applied after the burn wound has been cooled. It should not be layered or wrapped around a limb, to avoid a tourniquet effect if swelling occurs. Avoid using ointments, lotions and powders in the immediate first aid period, as they can alter the wound's appearance and hinder the assessment of burn depth.

CLASSIFICATION OF BURNS

The severity of a burn is typically determined by two main factors: its depth (how deeply it penetrates the layers of skin) and its extent (how much total body surface area it covers). Burn classification is based on these factors, which are crucial for deciding the appropriate treatment and predicting the prognosis.

DEPTH

The depth of a burn will affect the rate at which the wound will heal on its own. The longer the healing process takes, the higher the risk of infection, scarring and loss of function. Various methods exist for classifying burn depth. In the UK, the most common method is to distinguish between partial-thickness and full-thickness skin destruction.

Superficial burns affect only the outer layer of the skin (epidermis), causing redness and pain, similar to a sunburn (Chadwick 2021).

Partial-thickness burns involve the epidermis and part of the dermis, while full-thickness burns destroy both the epidermis and the entire dermis. Superficial partial-thickness burns involve the epidermis and part of the dermis, leading to blistering, swelling and intense pain as the sensory nerve endings are exposed to the air. Deep partial-thickness burns extend deeper into the dermis, potentially causing white or charred skin and more severe pain.

Full-thickness burns penetrate through the dermis and affect deeper tissues; they may also involve deeper structures such as fat, muscle and bone. These burns can appear white, brown or black and may be painless due to nerve damage.

EXTENT

The extent of burns is calculated as a percentage of total body surface area affected. This assessment is crucial for treatment planning, particularly for determining the need for fluid resuscitation.

When burns occur, there is an inflammatory response that leads to increased blood flow to the area (hyperaemia) and the movement of fluids from the intravascular to interstitial compartments. If this happens in a small area, covering less than 5% of the body surface, the effects are localised. However, when a larger portion of the body surface is injured (or traumatised), there is a massive fluid shift into the tissues that occurs, resulting in a significant reduction in circulating volume. It is generally accepted that children with burns covering more than 10% of their body surface area and adults with burns covering more than 15% will experience hypovolaemic shock unless there is prompt intravenous fluid replacement (McCahill 2019).

To estimate the percentage of body surface affected, the simplest and most easily remembered method is the long-established 'rule of nines' that was introduced by Wallace in 1951 (see Figure 6.1). According to this method, the head and each upper limb account for 9%, while the anterior trunk, posterior trunk and each lower limb account for 18% each. The remaining 1% is usually assigned to the perineum (Lee 2022).

Lee (2022) notes that it is important to remember that differences exist between adults and children when estimating burns. The rule of nines should not be used for estimating burn percentage in young children. This tool does not allow for the different proportions of head and lower limbs in infants and toddlers. The Lund and Browder chart is a recognised tool that is used to calculate the percentage of total body surface in children (see Figure 6.2).

McCahill (2019) suggests that a rapid approximation of the percentage can be made by using the palmar aspect of the patient's hand (with fingers together) as 1% of the body surface area.

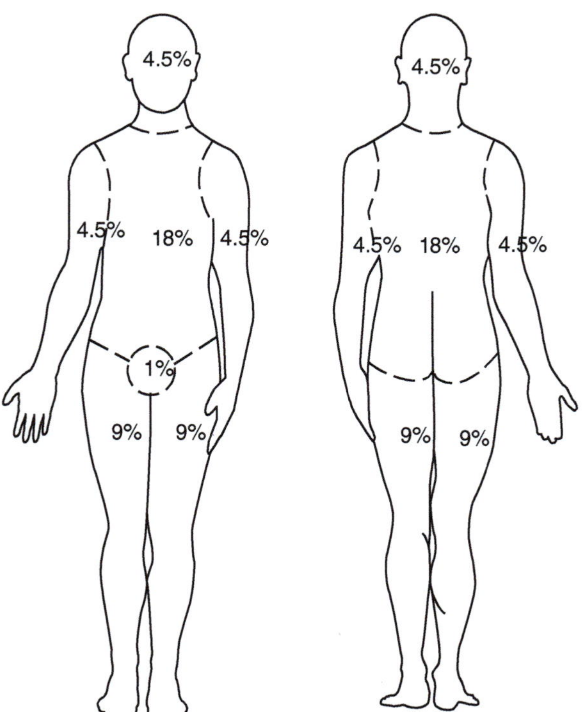

FIGURE 6.1 Wallace's rule of nines

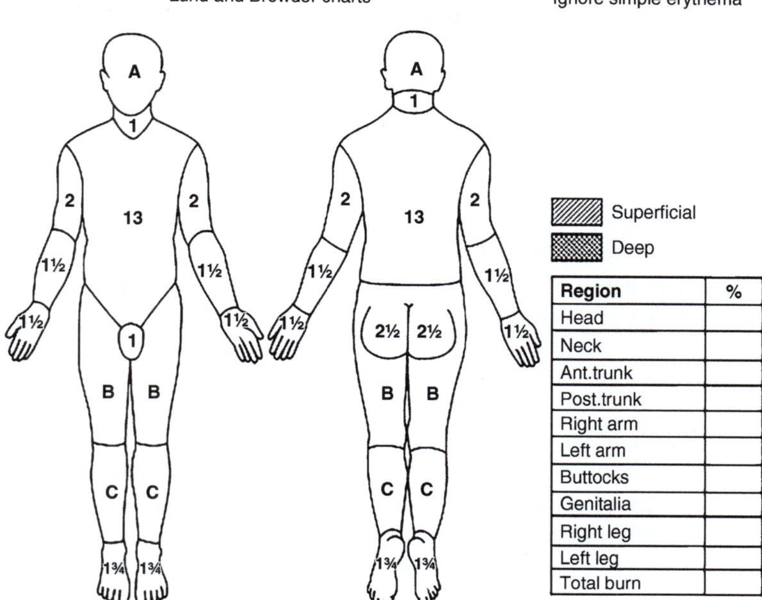

Region	%
Head	
Neck	
Ant.trunk	
Post.trunk	
Right arm	
Left arm	
Buttocks	
Genitalia	
Right leg	
Left leg	
Total burn	

Relative percentage of body surface area affected by growth

Area	Age 0	1	5	10	15	Adult
A = ½ of head	9½	8½	6½	5½	4½	3½
B = ½ of one thigh	2¾	3¼	4	4½	4½	4¾
C = ½ of one leg	2½	2½	2¾	3	3¼	3½

FIGURE 6.2 Lund and Browder burns assessment tool

COMPLICATIONS AND ASSOCIATED PROBLEMS

Burn injuries can cause several complications, including:

- Hypovolaemic shock: Significant fluid loss from severe burns can decrease blood volume, leading to shock and necessitating immediate fluid resuscitation.

- Inhalation injury: Burns to the respiratory tract from inhaling smoke or toxic fumes can lead to serious respiratory issues.

- Infection: Damaged skin loses its protective barrier, increasing the risk of bacterial infections.

- Scarring and contractures: Deep burns can result in extensive scarring and contractures, which are tightened areas of skin that can limit movement and function. Additionally, individuals who experience deep burns may face significant psychological issues, including post-traumatic stress disorder, anxiety, depression and body image concerns.

PATHOPHYSIOLOGICAL CHANGES ASSOCIATED WITH BURNS

Understanding the multiple functions of the skin and its roles in homeostasis can help to make it easier to understand the sequelae of a burn injury (see Chapter 1 of this book). Burn injuries initiate a complex and multifaceted series of pathophysiological changes that lead to a cascade of changes in the body, impacting multiple systems occurring within the first few hours after the event (Martin, Cheek, and Morris 2019). These changes can range from local tissue damage to systemic responses that impact various organs. Pathophysiological changes associated with burns include local and systemic responses, metabolic changes, alterations in immune function and complications related to wound healing.

LOCAL TISSUE DAMAGE

Burn injuries primarily result from thermal damage, leading to coagulation of proteins and cellular necrosis. The depth of tissue destruction depends on the temperature of the heat source and the duration of exposure.

INFLAMMATORY RESPONSE

When burn injuries occur, they trigger the body's immune system to release certain proteins called cytokines, specifically tumour necrosis factor-alpha (TNF-α), interleukin-1 (IL-1) and interleukin-6 (IL-6). These cytokines not only play a key role in the inflammatory response, which is the body's natural reaction to injury or infection, but can also exacerbate tissue damage if the inflammatory response becomes excessive or uncontrolled.

INCREASED VASCULAR PERMEABILITY

In the case of burns, increased vascular permeability refers to the condition where the blood vessels in the affected area become more permeable or 'leaky'. Normally, blood vessels maintain a tight barrier that regulates the movement of fluids, proteins and other substances between the bloodstream and surrounding tissues. When vascular permeability increases due to a burn injury:

- The walls of the blood vessels become more porous, allowing fluids, proteins and other components of blood to escape from the bloodstream and enter the surrounding interstitial space (the space between cells in the tissue).

- This escape of fluids into the interstitial space results in oedema. Oedema occurs because the fluid accumulates in the tissues, leading to increased volume and pressure in the affected area.

The process of increased vascular permeability and subsequent oedema can have several implications in burn injuries:

- The accumulation of fluid causes noticeable swelling in the burned area, which can be painful and restrict movement, especially if the burn is on a limb or near a joint.

- The increased pressure from the fluid accumulation can impair blood flow to the affected and surrounding tissues, leading to further tissue damage and delayed healing.

- In severe cases, the swelling can be so intense that it creates excessive pressure within muscle compartments, leading to compartment syndrome, a serious condition that can compromise circulation and nerve function.

- The loss of fluids and proteins from the vascular system into the tissues reduces the overall blood volume and can lead to hypovolaemia (a decrease in the volume of circulating blood). This can result in shock, a critical condition requiring immediate medical intervention.

Neutrophils and macrophages migrate to the injury site, releasing reactive oxygen species and enzymes that can further damage tissues.

VASCULAR CHANGES

The increased capillary permeability results in significant fluid loss from the vascular space into the interstitial space. This fluid shift can lead to:

- Hypovolaemic shock: due to significant loss of intravascular volume, resulting in decreased cardiac output and tissue perfusion.

- Compartment syndrome: increased tissue pressure from oedema can compromise blood flow, leading to tissue ischaemia and necrosis.

SYSTEMIC EFFECTS

Severe burns can induce systemic inflammatory response syndrome, characterised by widespread inflammation that affects the entire body. This can progress to multiple organ dysfunction syndrome, a severe condition involving the failure of two or more organ systems, often leading to death. Inhalation injuries can occur alongside burns, particularly in fire incidents, causing damage to the airways and lungs, leading to conditions such as acute respiratory distress syndrome.

METABOLIC CHANGES

People with burns can experience a significant increase in metabolic rate, which leads to elevated caloric and protein needs due to enhanced catabolism. Protein catabolism leads to the breakdown of muscle tissue, contributing to weakness and delayed recovery (muscle wasting). Challenges in meeting increased nutritional demands can impair wound healing and immune function.

IMMUNE SUPPRESSION

Burns compromise the immune system, which can make patients vulnerable to infections. Factors contributing to this include the loss of skin barrier; the primary defence against pathogens is compromised in burns. Burn injuries can significantly result in immune cell dysfunction and altered cytokine production. These changes increase the risk of infections by impairing the body's ability to defend against pathogens and by creating an environment that supports microbial growth.

FLUID AND ELECTROLYTE IMBALANCE

This refers to the significant disturbances in the body's normal fluid and electrolyte levels that occur as a result of burn injuries. These imbalances can have serious consequences if they are not managed appropriately. Fluid and electrolyte imbalance is a key issue in the management of burn injuries due to the significant fluid shifts and losses associated with the damage. Close monitoring and correction of electrolyte imbalances, such as sodium and potassium, is crucial to prevent complications, for example, arrhythmias and renal failure.

WOUND HEALING

Stages of healing:

- Inflammatory phase: characterised by haemostasis and inflammation, lasting a few days.

- Proliferative phase: involves tissue regeneration and collagen deposition, lasting weeks.

- Maturation phase: final remodelling of the wound, which can last months to years.

Extensive burns can lead to hypertrophic scars (thick, raised scars that form because of an overactive healing process) and contractures (occurring when the skin and underlying tissues tighten excessively as they heal from a burn, leading to restricted movement), impairing function and appearance. Surgical interventions such as skin grafts and physiotherapy are often required.

LONG-TERM COMPLICATIONS

There are a number of long-term complications associated with burns, including:

- Chronic/persistent pain due to nerve damage and scarring.

- Burn injuries can lead to significant emotional and psychological distress, requiring mental health support and counselling (McGovern, Puxty, and Paton 2022).

- Severe burns, especially those involving joints and limbs, can lead to long-term disability and reduced quality of life.

Managing burn injuries requires a multidisciplinary approach addressing the immediate physiological needs, such as fluid resuscitation and infection control, as well as long-term rehabilitation to support recovery and improve outcomes. Early intervention, continuous monitoring and tailored therapeutic strategies are essential in mitigating the extensive pathophysiological impacts of burns.

EPIDEMIOLOGY

Burn injuries in the UK impact significantly on affected individuals and the healthcare system. Understanding the epidemiology helps in formulating targeted prevention strategies, improving treatment protocols and enhancing rehabilitation services to reduce the incidence and severity of burns and improve outcomes for burn victims.

The exact prevalence of burn injuries is unknown as some people will self-treat and do not seek medical attention. It is estimated that there are approximately 10 000 hospital admissions and 300 major burns in adults requiring fluid resuscitation in England and Wales per year. In Scotland, there is an incidence of 500 burn injury admissions per year, of which 5% of these are major burns (see McCann, Watson, and Barnes 2022). The most common injury leading to hospital admission is scalds, while flame injuries are the primary cause of major burns (International Burn Injury Database 2020). There has been a downwards trend in burn incidence and injury severity (Smolle et al. 2017)

The majority of burn injuries happen accidentally, either at home or in the workplace. However, when burns are caused intentionally, through acts of self-harm, assaults or deliberate fires, these incidents are more likely to lead to severe or major burns (Peck 2012).

The epidemiology of burns provides the foundational data and insights that are necessary to understand who is most at risk and why burns occur. This information is key for conducting thorough risk assessments, which aim to prevent burns and mitigate their impact. By identifying patterns and causes, both fields work together to enhance burn prevention, improve safety measures and ultimately reduce the incidence and severity of burn injuries.

RISK FACTORS

The epidemiology of burns and the assessment of burn risks are interconnected. Understanding the risk factors that are associated with burns is essential for effective prevention, resource allocation, treatment, education, research and economic efficiency. It enables the development of targeted strategies that can significantly reduce the incidence and severity of burn injuries, ultimately improving public health and safety. See Table 6.1 for risk factors associated with burns.

Table 6.1 Risk factors associated with burns

Risk factor	Discussion
Gender	Women have slightly higher rates of death from burns compared to men. Unlike most types of injuries where men generally have higher rates of incidence, the death rates from burn injuries are slightly higher for women. Typically, men tend to be injured more frequently across various types of incidents, but in the specific case of burn-related fatalities, women are more affected.
	The higher risk for women is associated with open fire cooking or unsafe cookstoves, which can cause their loose clothing to catch fire. Open flames used for heating and lighting also pose risks, and self-harm and domestic violence are also factors.
Age	In addition to adult women, children are especially susceptible to burns. Burns rank as the fifth most frequent cause of non-fatal childhood injuries. Insufficient adult supervision represents a significant risk factor, yet a notable portion of burn injuries in children arise from non-accidental injury.
	Elderly people are at higher risk due to their vulnerability to accidents and slower reaction times.
Regional factors	Important regional differences in burn rates exist.
	Children under five years of age in the World Health Organization (WHO) African Region have over two times the incidence of burn deaths than those children under five years of age worldwide.
	Boys under five years of age living in low- and middle-income countries of the WHO Eastern Mediterranean Region are almost twice as likely to die from burns as boys living in the WHO European Region.
	The incidence of burn injuries requiring medical care is nearly 20 times higher in the WHO Western Pacific Region than in the WHO Region of the Americas.
Socioeconomic factors	Those people living in low- and middle-income countries are at higher risk for burns than those living in high-income countries. Within all countries, however, burn risk correlates with socioeconomic status.

(Continued)

Table 6.1 (*Continued*)

Risk factor	Discussion
Other risk factors	There are a number of other risk factors for burns, including: • Lack of education and awareness • Occupations that have an increased exposure to fire • Poverty, overcrowding and lack of effective safety measures • Assigning young girls to household duties such as cooking and caring for young children • Pre-existing medical conditions, including epilepsy, peripheral neuropathy and physical and cognitive disabilities • Alcohol misuse and smoking • Injuries are more common in patients with pre-existing psychiatric diagnoses • Easy access to chemicals that are used for assault (such as in acid violence attacks) • Use of kerosene (paraffin) as a fuel source for non-electric domestic appliances • Insufficient safety measures in place for liquefied petroleum gas and electricity

Source: Adapted from WHO (2023), McCann, Watson, and Barnes (2022), McGovern, Puxty, and Paton (2022) and Jordan et al. (2022).

Burn injuries can be prevented and efforts to reduce their occurrence primarily emphasise increasing awareness, providing education and implementing health and safety regulations. By taking thorough and inclusive actions to address the various factors that contribute to burn injuries, it is possible to reduce the overall impact and frequency of burns. This comprehensive approach aims not only to prevent burns but also to improve overall safety and well-being in communities. Identifying, understanding and effectively mitigating these risk factors, individuals and communities can create safer environments and reduce the occurrence of burn-related injuries and their associated negative consequences.

CLINICAL PRESENTATION

The clinical presentation of burns varies depending on factors such as the depth and extent of the injury, location and associated symptoms. Prompt and accurate assessment of burns is essential for determining the appropriate treatment and minimising complications. Understanding the clinical features of burns helps in the provision of comprehensive care and support to patients with burn injuries. See Table 6.2 for a summary of burn depth.

CLINICAL INVESTIGATIONS AND DIAGNOSIS

Diagnosing a burn primarily involves a thorough clinical assessment. There are several clinical investigations that can aid in evaluating the severity and extent of the injury, potential complications and the patient's overall condition. A comprehensive approach ensures that all aspects of the patient's health are considered, facilitating effective and tailored treatment.

Table 6.2 A summary of burn depth

Depth of burn	Skin layers affected
Superficial epidermal (such as sunburn) Not usually life-threatening	The epidermis is affected, but the dermis is intact.
Superficial dermal (partial thickness)	Superficial dermal (partial thickness).
	The epidermis and the upper and deeper layers of the dermis are involved, but not underlying subcutaneous tissues. The area may be wet due to interstitial fluid loss.
Full thickness	The burn penetrates all skin layers, reaching the subcutaneous tissues. In severe cases, it may extend further into muscle and bone. Scaring is likely.

Source: Adapted from McCahill (2019); Douglas and Ford (2017).

CLINICAL ASSESSMENT

The clinical assessment of burns is a critical step in diagnosing and formulating a treatment plan for burn patients. This comprehensive evaluation involves several key components, each designed to determine the severity, extent and potential complications of the burn injury. A detailed clinical assessment allows healthcare providers to deliver targeted and effective care, optimising patient outcomes.

VISUAL EXAMINATION

The initial step in the clinical assessment is a thorough visual examination of the burn wounds. Healthcare providers assess the depth of the burns.

VITAL SIGNS MONITORING

Monitoring vital signs is essential to assess the patient's overall stability and detect signs of systemic involvement.

PATIENT HISTORY

A detailed patient history is taken to understand the context of the burn injury. Important aspects include:

- Cause of the burn

- Environment of the incident

- Pre-existing medical conditions

- Medications

LABORATORY INVESTIGATIONS

Laboratory tests are conducted to provide further insight into the patient's condition and guide treatment decisions.

IMAGING STUDIES

Imaging studies, such as chest X-rays, may be performed to identify inhalation injuries, pulmonary complications such as pneumonia or acute respiratory distress syndrome and to assess for fluid overload. In more severe cases, a CT scan might be used to allow detailed images of the chest, abdomen or head to identify internal injuries or complications.

Integrating these components into a thorough clinical assessment can help to accurately diagnose the severity of burn injuries, identify potential complications and develop a comprehensive, individualised treatment plan. This approach is essential for optimising patient outcomes and facilitating effective, targeted care for burn victims.

MANAGEMENT

Immediate first aid is provided to the person with burns. All major burns are traumatic injuries and should be treated according to the principles associated with advanced trauma life support. Treatment recommendations are provided by the International Society for Burn Injuries (2016, 2018) and National Institute for Health and Care Excellence (2012, 2016). Table 6.3 provides an overview of the management of burn patients.

By following the guidelines issued, those who offer care and support to people with burns can effectively manage issues these patients face, promote healing, prevent complications and improve overall care outcomes.

Table 6.3 An overview of key aspects of the management of burn patients

Approach	Discussion
Initial assessment and stabilisation	Primary survey:
	Airway: Assess for airway patency. Observe for signs of inhalation injury (e.g. soot in the mouth/nose, singed nasal hairs, hoarseness, stridor). Secure the airway if there is any doubt.
	Breathing: Assess breathing. Administer oxygen and monitor for signs of respiratory distress.
	Circulation: Evaluate circulation. Establish intravenous access with large-bore cannulae and begin fluid resuscitation. Monitor for signs of shock.
	Disability: Assess neurological status using the AVPU scale (alert, responds to voice, responds to pain, unresponsive) or Glasgow Coma Scale.
	Exposure: Remove all clothing and jewellery to prevent further tissue damage. Keep the patient warm to prevent hypothermia.
	Secondary survey:
	Undertake a head-to-toe examination to identify all injuries.
	Determine burn depth and extent using the rule of nines, Lund–Browder chart or the patient's palm.
Fluid resuscitation	For burns greater than 15–20% of the total body surface, initiate fluid resuscitation to prevent burn shock. There are a number of formulae available, for example, Parkland, Muir or Barclay formulae. The use of a volumetric intravenous pump provides accuracy for infusion of volumes of fluid required in each period, which may be very large.

Approach	Discussion
	Monitor urine output via urinary catheter (0.5 mL/kg/h) as a guide to adequate resuscitation.
	There may be a reduction in gastrointestinal tract perfusion that results from hypovolaemia. As such, it is necessary, initially, to restrict the volume of oral fluids until it has been established that there is no nausea or vomiting. A nasogastric tube is passed and drained freely or is aspirated hourly if there is vomiting prior to small amounts of water being given.
Pain management	Administer pain relief, commencing with intravenous opioids (e.g. morphine, fentanyl) as required via infusion pump, give an initial dose first.
	Use adjunctive medications (e.g. anxiolytics) for anxiety and pain management.
	If the patient is in shock, the intramuscular route is not used, as the medication will not be absorbed due to peripheral vasoconstriction.
Wound care	The depth of the burn is estimated and charted, noting its position and extent. Colour photographs are often taken for recording purposes as well as being a baseline record of wound appearance and distribution. While the wounds are exposed, swabs can be taken for bacteriological examination from each wound site, e.g. right hand, left hand, chest and neck. This can reduce the potential of wound contamination, discomfort and the possible loss of dignity experienced by the patient during repeated removal of the dressings. The initial wound swabs may reveal no bacteriological contamination; they do, however, provide a useful baseline for further monitoring. Initially, wounds are then covered with a temporary dressing. A specific care regimen will be decided upon once the patient's condition has been stabilised.
	Debridement of any necrotic tissue may be required and the application of topical antimicrobial (e.g. silver sulfadiazine, mafenide acetate).
	Dressings are used to maintain a moist wound environment and to prevent infection.
	Escharotomies or fasciotomies may be necessary for circumferential burns to prevent compartment syndrome.
	Escharotomies: This is a surgical procedure that involves making incisions through the eschar (the thick, leathery, dead tissue that forms on the surface of the skin after a severe burn). This procedure is performed to relieve pressure and restore blood flow.
	Fasciotomies: This is another surgical procedure that involves cutting the fascia (the connective tissue surrounding muscles) to relieve pressure and improve circulation. This is more invasive than an escharotomy and is done when deeper structures are affected.
	Circumferential burns: These are burns that encircle a body part, such as an arm, leg or torso. Because the skin and underlying tissues become tight and inflexible, these burns can create a constricting band.
	Compartment syndrome: This is a serious condition that occurs when pressure within the muscles builds to dangerous levels, decreasing blood flow and potentially leading to muscle and nerve damage. This can be caused by circumferential burns due to the swelling and tightness they cause.
	Specialist advice is required for wound care in relation to burns.

(Continued)

Table 6.3 (*Continued*)

Approach	Discussion
Infection prevention and control	Apply aseptic techniques during wound care.
	Administer tetanus prophylaxis.
	Consider systemic antibiotics for patients with signs of infection or inhalation injury.
Nutritional support	Burns patients have increased metabolic demands. Start enteral nutrition early to meet these needs.
	High-calorie, high-protein diets are essential for healing.
Rehabilitation and psychological support	Physical therapy and occupational therapy should be initiated early to prevent contractures and maintain function.
	Provide psychological support to address the emotional and mental impact of burns.
Monitoring and follow-up	Monitor vital signs and laboratory values (e.g. electrolytes, renal function) closely.
	Pulse:
	If the patient is shocked, the pulse will be rapid and weak. This, combined with generalised oedema, can make manual counting very difficult and mechanical aids are normally used.
	Blood pressure:
	It is not usual practice to record blood pressure if all four limbs have been burned. Indeed, this practice is often avoided in such cases. If one limb is unaffected, it is considered more important to ensure effective intravenous access and fluid replacement as opposed to repeatedly constricting the vessels with a blood pressure cuff.
	The routine measurement of central venous pressure or arterial pressure is not recommended as there is a risk of systemic infection related to such invasive techniques, particularly if the site of entry of the catheter is close to the burn wound.
	Temperature:
	A reliable indicator of the state of peripheral perfusion is the difference between the core and shell temperatures. Temperature monitoring is usually facilitated by the use of thermistor probes as opposed to repeated insertion of a rectal thermometer. Measuring the core temperature will indicate a trend towards hyperpyrexia or hypothermia.
	Adjust fluid resuscitation based on clinical response and urine output.
	Wounds are regularly reassessed and dressings and treatments adjusted as needed according to local policy and protocol.
Infection prevention and control	As there are large areas of skin accompanied by exudate and necrotic tissue, burn wounds rapidly become colonised with bacteria, it is essential that meticulous attention is paid to the prevention of cross-infection. The patient should be cared for in a single room where possible and standard infection control precautions implemented. Personal protective equipment must be used whenever the patient is cared for and local policy and procedure must be adhered to.

Approach	Discussion
Psychological effects of burn injuries	Burn injuries can have profound psychological impact including post-traumatic stress disorder, depression and anxiety. Psychological support and counselling are integral parts of the recovery process to address these issues.
	The disfigurement and impaired function resulting from wound contracture and scar formation are major sequelae of burn injuries, resulting in distress and psychological problems for the patient and their family/carers.
	Care provision must be focused on the individual, with the patient at the centre of all that is done. Many patients voice their relief at being alive in the immediate period after the accident; however, as the implications of their injury become apparent, their emotions and behaviour can begin to change.

Source: Adapted from McCahill (2019).

HEALTH TEACHING

Burn prevention and health education are the most effective ways of decreasing burn mortality and morbidity. Health teaching for patients with burns is crucial to ensure proper healing, prevent complications and support overall recovery.

WOUND CARE

The patient is given information and advice regarding wound care. If appropriate, offer advice on dressing changes, including hand hygiene and using sterile techniques. Explain signs of infection to be aware of, such as increased redness, swelling, pus or a foul odour. Emphasise the importance of keeping the wound area clean and dry and adhere to any instructions provided regarding wound care.

PAIN MANAGEMENT

Explain to the patient the importance of taking prescribed pain medications as directed and discuss any potential side effects and when to contact a healthcare provider.

INFECTION PREVENTION

Stress the importance of regular handwashing before touching the wound or changing dressings. Offer advice on maintaining a clean environment to minimise infection risk.

NUTRITION AND HYDRATION

Explain the need for a high-protein, high-calorie diet to support wound healing. Suggest foods rich in vitamins and minerals, especially vitamins A and C and zinc. Encourage adequate fluid intake to support overall health and healing.

PHYSICAL ACTIVITY AND REHABILITATION

Teach range-of-movement exercises to prevent stiffness and promote mobility. Explain the importance of physiotherapy and adherence to prescribed exercise routines.

SCAR MANAGEMENT

The use of compression garments is essential to minimise scarring and support the healing process for burn patients. These garments help reduce hypertrophic scarring and prevent the formation of contractures by applying consistent pressure to the affected areas. To ensure patients benefit fully from this treatment, detailed advice should be provided to reinforce the instructions given by specialist healthcare practitioners.

PSYCHOLOGICAL SUPPORT

Burn injuries can have a profound psychological impact on patients, affecting their emotional well-being and mental health. Comprehensive psychological support is crucial for their recovery and long-term adjustment. This support encompasses mental health awareness, access to counselling and information about support groups.

FOLLOW-UP CARE

Stress the importance of attending all follow-up appointments for ongoing assessment and care and report any concerns to their healthcare provider.

SELF-CARE AND LIFESTYLE ADJUSTMENTS

Patients with burns may need to make several self-care and lifestyle adjustments to support their healing and prevent complications.

Burn-injured skin is highly sensitive to ultraviolet (UV) radiation from the sun. Protecting these areas is crucial to prevent further damage, hyperpigmentation and an increased risk of skin cancer. Advise patients to use a broad-spectrum sunscreen with a high sun protection factor (SPF), preferably SPF 30 or higher. Sunscreen is applied generously to all healed burn areas and should be reapplied every two hours or more frequently if swimming or sweating.

Recommend wearing protective clothing, such as long sleeves, pants and wide-brimmed hats, to shield healed burn areas from direct sun exposure. Suggest the use of clothing made from fabrics that offer UV protection.

Avoiding peak sun hours. Seek shade whenever possible if the person needs to be outdoors during these hours.

Certain substances, such as tobacco and alcohol, can significantly impair the healing process and overall health of people with burns. Smoking reduces blood flow, delays healing and increases the risk of infections and complications. Provide information on smoking cessation programmes, support groups and medications that can assist in stopping smoking.

Alcohol has the potential to impair immune function, dehydrate the body and interfere with the healing process. Encourage patients to limit alcohol intake and suggest healthier alternatives, such as non-alcoholic beverages or water.

Addressing the health teaching needs of people with burns can empower them to manage their care effectively, promote healing and reduce the risk of complications.

CONCLUSION

Burn injuries require a comprehensive and multidisciplinary approach to treatment and rehabilitation. Understanding the classification, potential complications and appropriate interventions is crucial for optimal recovery and minimising long-term impacts on the patient's health and quality of life. The management of burns involves immediate medical care, ongoing wound treatment, rehabilitation and psychological support to ensure the best possible outcomes.

Burns are injuries of skin or other tissue caused by thermal, radiation, chemical or electrical contact. Burns are classified by depth (superficial and deep partial-thickness and full-thickness) and percentage of total body surface area involved. Complications and associated problems include hypovolaemic shock, inhalation injury, infection, scarring and contractures. Patients with large burns (20% total body surface area) require fluid resuscitation. Treatments for burn wounds include topical antibacterials, regular cleansing, elevation and sometimes skin grafting. Intensive rehabilitation, consisting of range-of-motion exercises and splinting, is often necessary as well psychological support is required.

GLOSSARY OF TERMS

Burn depth: The classification of burns based on how deeply the skin is affected: superficial, partial-thickness or full-thickness.

Contractures: Tightened areas of skin that can develop as burn wounds heal, potentially limiting movement and function.

Debridement: The medical removal of dead, damaged or infected tissue to improve the healing potential of the remaining healthy tissue.

Eschar: A piece of dead tissue that is cast off from the surface of the skin, particularly after a burn injury.

Escharotomy: A surgical procedure to cut through the eschar to relieve pressure and improve blood flow to the area beneath, often necessary in severe burns.

Grafting: The surgical procedure of transplanting skin or other tissues to cover and heal a burn wound.

Inhalation injury: Damage to the respiratory tract or lungs caused by inhaling smoke, chemicals or hot air, which can complicate burn injuries.

Infection: The invasion and multiplication of microorganisms in body tissues, which can be a serious complication of burns.

Lund and Browder chart: A tool used to estimate the total body surface area affected by burns, providing a more detailed assessment than the rule of nines, particularly for children.

Nutritional support: Ensuring adequate intake of calories, proteins and nutrients essential for wound healing and recovery in burn patients.

Partial-thickness burn: A burn that affects the epidermis and part of the dermis, characterised by redness, blistering and significant pain.

Rule of nines: A quick method to estimate the total body surface area affected by burns, dividing the body into sections that represent 9% (or multiples of 9%) of the total area.

Scarring: The formation of fibrous tissue as a wound heals, which can be extensive in burn injuries.

Superficial burn: A burn affecting only the outer layer of the skin (epidermis), typically causing redness and pain without blistering.

Total body surface area: The percentage of the body affected by burns, important for determining the severity of the injury and guiding treatment.

MULTIPLE CHOICE QUESTIONS

1. Which of the following is the primary purpose of an escharotomy in burn patients?
   a) To improve cosmetic appearance
   b) To relieve pressure and restore circulation
   c) To prevent infection
   d) To reduce pain

2. What is the rule of nines used for in burn management?
   a) Estimating the depth of a burn
   b) Calculating the amount of fluid resuscitation needed
   c) Assessing the total body surface area affected by burns
   d) Determining the need for surgery

3. Which type of burn is characterised by damage that extends through the entire dermis and potentially deeper tissues?
   a) Superficial burn
   b) Partial-thickness burn
   c) Full-thickness burn
   d) First-degree burn

4. Which of the following is NOT a common complication of severe burns?
   a) Hypovolaemic shock
   b) Hyperglycaemia
   c) Infection
   d) Contractures

5. What is the primary function of compression garments in burn care?
   a) To prevent infection
   b) To reduce scarring
   c) To control pain
   d) To improve circulation

6. Which sign is an indication of inhalation injury in a burn patient?
   a) Dry, pale skin
   b) Singed nasal hairs
   c) Blistering on the skin
   d) Decreased urine output

7. What type of burn injury involves only the epidermis and presents with redness and pain, but no blisters?
   a) First-degree burn
   b) Second-degree burn
   c) Third-degree burn
   d) Fourth-degree burn

8. What is the purpose of using a Lund and Browder chart in burn assessment?
   a) To estimate the depth of a burn
   b) To calculate the total body surface area affected
   c) To determine the need for surgery
   d) To assess for inhalation injury

9. What is the initial step in the management of chemical burns?
   a) Applying antibiotic ointment
   b) Cooling the burn with ice
   c) Irrigating the area with copious amounts of water
   d) Covering the burn with a sterile dressing

10. In burn care, what does debridement involve?
   a) Covering the wound with a sterile dressing
   b) Removing dead or damaged tissue
   c) Applying antibiotic ointment
   d) Cooling the burn with ice

REFERENCES

British Burn Association (2018). First aid clinical practice guidelines. https://www.britishburnassociation.org/wp-content/uploads/2017/06/BBA-First-Aid-Guideline-24.9.18.pdf (accessed May 2024).

Chadwick, A. L. (2021). Basic first aid (Chapter 18). In: *The Nursing Associate's Handbook of Clinical Skills* (ed. I. Peate). Oxford: Wiley.

Douglas, H.E. and Ford, W. (2017). Burns dressings. *Australian Family Practitioners* 46 (3): 94–97.

Huang, S.W., Yeh, F.C., Ji, Y.R. et al. (2021). Chitosan-based hydrogels to treat hydrofluoric acid burns and prevent infection. *Drug Delivery and Translational Research* 11. 1532–1544.

International Burn Injury Database (2020). Adult resuscitation burns 2019/20 and causation covering 2019 to 2020 inclusive. England: Ad hoc report request in McCann, C., Watson, A., and Barnes, D. (2022) Major burns: Part 1. Epidemiology, pathophysiology and initial management. *British Journal of Anaesthesia Education* 22 (3): 94–103. doi: 10.1016/j.bjae.2021.10.001. 2022.

International Society for Burn Injuries (2016). ISBI practice guidelines for burn care. *Burns* 42 (5): 953–1021.

International Society for Burn Injuries (2018). ISBI practice guidelines for burn care, Part 2. *Burns* 44 (7): 1617–1706.

Jordan, K.C., Di Gennaro, J.L., von Saint André-von, Arnim. et al. (2022). Global trends in pediatric burn injuries and care capacity from the World Health Organization global burn registry. *Frontiers in Pediatric* 10. 954995. doi: 10.3389/fped.2022.954995.

Lee, N. (2022). Burn care within a critical care setting (Chapter 28). In: *Fundamentals of Critical Care* (ed. I. Peate and B. Hill). Oxford: Wiley.

Martin, L.L., Cheek, D.J., and Morris, S.E. (2019). Shock, multiple organ dysfunction syndrome, and burns in adults (Chapter 49). In: *Pathophysiology. The Biologic Basis for Disease in Adults and Children*, 8e (ed. K.L. Mc. Cance, and S. E. Huether). St Louis: Elsevier.

McCahill, B. (2019). Nursing the patient with burns (Chapter 28). In: *Alexander's Nursing Practice*, 5e (ed. I. Peate). London: Elsevier.

McCann, C., Watson, A., and Barnes, D. (2022). Major burns: Part 1. Epidemiology, pathophysiology and initial management. *British Journal of Anaesthesia Education* 22 (3): 94–103. doi: 10.1016/j.bjae.2021.10.001.

McGovern, C., Puxty, K., and Paton, L. (2022). Major burns: Part 2. Anaesthesia, intensive care and pain management. *British Journal of Anaesthesia Education* 22 (4): 138–145. doi: 10.1016/j.bjae.2022.01.001.

Mclure, M., Macneil, F., Wood, F.M. et al. (2021). A rapid review of burns first aid guidelines: is there consistency across international guidelines? *Cureus* 13 (6): e15779. doi: 10.7759/cureus.15779.

National Institute for Health and Care Excellence (2012). National burn care referral guidance. https://www.britishburnassociation.org/wp-content/uploads/2018/02/National-Burn-Care-Referral-Guidance-2012.pdf (accessed June 2024).

National Institute for Health and Care Excellence (2016). Mersey burns for calculating fluid resuscitation volume when managing burns.

https://www.nice.org.uk/advice/mib58/resources/mersey-burns-for-calculating-fluid-resuscitation-volume-when-managing-burns-pdf-63499233245893 (accessed June 2024).

Peck, M.D. (2012). Epidemiology of burns throughout the world: Part II. Intentional burns in adults. *Burns* 38 (5): 630–637.

Smolle, C., Cambiaso-Daniel, J., Forbes, A.A. et al. (2017). Recent trends in burn epidemiology worldwide: a systematic review. *Burns* 43 (2): 249–257.

Wright, E.H., Harris, A.L., and Furniss, D. (2015). Cooling of burns: mechanisms and models. *Burns* 41. 82–889.

World Health Organization (2023). Burns. https://www.who.int/news-room/fact-sheets/detail/burns (accessed May 2024).

Herpes Zoster

HERPES INFECTION

Once acquired, all herpes virus infections are lifelong. As such, the disease is caused by primary infection but also secondary reactivation, the latter typically occurring when immunity wanes (as a result of immunosuppression or simply ageing). Herpes is a general term used to describe infections caused by the herpes simplex virus (HSV). Oral herpes, typically caused by HSV-1, presents as cold sores on or in the mouth. Genital herpes, a sexually transmitted infection, is usually caused by HSV-2. Herpes is spread by skin contact with the virus. There is no cure, but outbreaks of both oral and genital herpes can be managed with antiviral therapy.

As of now, eight members of the herpesvirus family have been identified. These viruses are found everywhere and are exceptionally adept as pathogens. The origin of the name lies in the Greek word 'herpein', which translates to 'to creep', indicative of the infections' tendency to be persistent, latent or recurrent (see Table 7.1).

PATHOPHYSIOLOGICAL CHANGES ASSOCIATED WITH HERPES ZOSTER

Herpes zoster is also known as shingles. Herpes zoster is caused by the varicella-zoster virus. After an attack of childhood chickenpox, the virus remains dormant in the dorsal root ganglia of the spinal cord and establishes a permanent latent infection but can be reactivated later in life to cause shingles. This means that varicella infection is a prerequisite for the development of shingles (UK Health Security Agency [UKHSA] 2024). The trigger factor is unknown, but the condition occurs in immunosuppressed people, stress and serious illness and commonly affects middle-aged and older people.

Once reactivated, varicella-zoster virus multiplies within host cells. The cells lyse and virus particles are released to invade other cells. The virus particles migrate along the sensory nerve fibres causing nerve damage and pain. Fluid-filled vesicles erupt along a thoracic and/ or cranial dermatome (an area of skin supplied by a nerve) with a characteristic one-sided (unilateral) band-like distribution of the sensory nerve. Pain and tenderness often precede the vesicular erosions and patients may have fever and feel unwell. As the vesicles crust over, the infective risk resolves over a period of two to three weeks.

REACTIVATION OF THE VIRUS

Latent virus: After chickenpox, the virus stays inactive in the sensory nerve cells (neurones) in the spinal cord or cranial nerves. Reactivation can occur when the immune system weakens due to ageing, stress, illness or immune-suppressing treatments.

SPREAD

Once reactivated, the virus then travels along the nerves to the skin. This process causes inflammation and damage to the nerves and skin causing pain. This is followed by the appearance of a rash. People with active lesions of shingles, particularly if they are immunocompromised, can transmit varicella-zoster virus to susceptible people to cause chickenpox. However, there is no evidence that shingles can be acquired from a person who has chickenpox.

Table 7.1 The herpesvirus family

Type	Discussion
Herpes simplex type 1	Herpes simplex type 1 (HSV-1) is a virus that primarily causes cold sores or fever blisters around the mouth and lips. It can also lead to other complications such as eye infections or encephalitis, which is an inflammation of the brain. HSV-1 is highly contagious and can be transmitted through direct contact with an infected person's saliva, skin or mucous membranes.
Herpes simplex type 2	Herpes simplex type 2 (HSV-2) is a virus that primarily causes genital herpes, which is a sexually transmitted infection characterised by outbreaks of sores or blisters in the genital area. It can also be transmitted to the mouth during oral sex, causing oral herpes. HSV-2 is highly contagious and can be spread through sexual contact with an infected person, even when they do not have visible sores.
Varicella-zoster virus	Varicella-zoster virus (VZV), also known as human herpesvirus 3 (HHV-3), is the virus responsible for causing chickenpox, a highly contagious disease typically occurring in childhood and characterised by an itchy rash and flu-like symptoms. After a person recovers from chickenpox, VZV remains dormant in the body's nerve tissues and can reactivate years later to cause shingles, a painful skin rash.
Epstein–Barr virus	Epstein–Barr virus (EBV), also known as human herpesvirus 4 (HHV-4), is one of the most common viruses in humans. It is best known for causing infectious mononucleosis, often referred to as 'mono' or 'the kissing disease'. EBV infection can lead to a range of symptoms, including fever, sore throat, swollen lymph nodes and fatigue. The virus is transmitted through bodily fluids, primarily saliva.
Cytomegalovirus	Cytomegalovirus (CMV), also known as human herpesvirus 5 (HHV-5), is a common virus that can infect almost anyone. Most people do not know they have CMV because it rarely causes problems in healthy people. However, it can cause disease in the newborn or in people with weakened immune systems. CMV is spread through close contact with body fluids and the infection can be silent or may cause symptoms similar to mononucleosis.
Herpesvirus type 6	Human herpesvirus 6 (HHV-6), also known as herpesvirus type 6, is a common virus that infects most people during childhood. It is associated with causing roseola, a mild illness characterised by a sudden high fever followed by a distinctive rash just as the fever breaks. HHV-6 can also reactivate later in life and has been studied for its potential association with various neurological conditions.
Herpesvirus type 7	Human herpesvirus 7 (HHV-7) is a virus similar to HHV-6 and is also commonly acquired during childhood. It is one of the possible causes of roseola, an illness that typically affects infants and young children, causing high fever and rash. For most people, infection with HHV-7 does not lead to significant illness, but like other herpesviruses, it remains in the body and can reactivate.
Kaposi's sarcoma herpesvirus	Kaposi's sarcoma herpesvirus (KSHV), also known as human herpesvirus 8 (HHV-8), is the virus that causes Kaposi's sarcoma, a cancer that forms masses in the skin, lymph nodes or other organs. KSHV is also associated with two other rare diseases: primary effusion lymphoma and multicentric Castleman's disease. It is transmitted through bodily fluids and is more common in people with weakened immune systems, such as those with HIV/AIDS.

IMMUNE RESPONSE AND INFLAMMATION

When the varicella-zoster virus reactivates and moves from the nerve ganglia to the skin, the body's immune system recognises the virus as a threat and mounts a defence against it. This immune response involves various immune cells and molecules that are designed to fight the virus. However, this response will also cause inflammation, which is a process that involves swelling, redness, heat and pain in the affected area. See Table 7.2 for an overview of the pathophysiological changes associated with herpes zoster.

In summary, as the immune system attempts to combat the reactivated varicella-zoster virus, this results in inflammation, which is responsible for the pain and the development of the characteristic rash and blisters that are associated with shingles.

Table 7.2 An overview of the pathophysiological changes associated with herpes zoster

Recognition of the virus

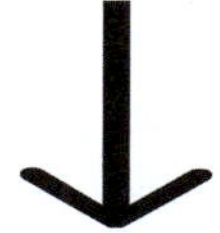

When varicella-zoster virus reactivates and travels along the nerves to the skin, the immune system detects the presence of the virus.

Immune response activation

Immune cells, including white blood cells such as T-cells and macrophages, are activated and travel to the site of the infection.

These cells release signalling molecules called cytokines and chemokines that help coordinate the immune response.

Inflammation

The cytokines and chemokines cause blood vessels in the affected area to dilate (widen) and become more permeable. This allows more immune cells to reach the site of the infection.

The increased blood flow and immune cell activity result in the characteristic signs of inflammation: redness, heat, swelling and pain.

Pain

The inflammation affects the nerves in the affected area, which can cause significant pain. This pain can be sharp, burning or throbbing and is often a primary symptom of shingles.

(Continued)

Table 7.2 (*Continued*)

Skin lesions

The immune response and the virus itself cause damage to the skin cells, leading to the formation of a rash. The rash typically starts as red patches, which then develop into fluid-filled blisters.

The blisters can break open, ooze fluid and then crust over as they heal.

Source: Adapted from Steinmann, Lampe, and Grosser (2023); Chowdhury, Katugampola, and Finlay (2019).

COMPLICATIONS

Some people, especially older adults, experience prolonged pain even after the rash heals, due to nerve damage; this is termed postherpetic neuralgia (Steinmann, Lampe, and Grosser 2023). The pain of postherpetic neuralgia may be sharp and intermittent or constant and may be debilitating. It may persist for months or years or permanently. In people with a weakened immune system, the virus can spread more widely, causing severe and widespread symptoms. This can lead to emotional distress, sleep disturbances and difficulty performing everyday tasks. Effective management requires a tailored approach that aims to reduce pain and improve the quality of life for those affected.

If the virus affects the nerves near the eye, it can lead to serious eye problems and potential vision loss (ophthalmic zoster). In some cases, varicella-zoster virus can spread to blood vessels, causing vasculopathy, which can lead to stroke. This is particularly a risk when shingles affect the ophthalmic distribution of the trigeminal nerve. Rarely, the virus can cause serious complications such as inflammation of the brain (encephalitis) or spinal cord (myelitis).

The immune system usually controls the reactivated virus over time, leading to healing of the skin lesions and a reduction in pain. An episode of shingles can boost the body's immunity to the virus, reducing the likelihood of future outbreaks.

TRANSMISSION

Varicella-zoster virus is transmitted from person to person through direct contact with the fluid from vesicular lesions or through inhalation of aerosols generated by these lesions. This mode of transmission occurs with acute varicella (chickenpox) or herpes zoster (shingles). Additionally, transmission can occur via infected respiratory secretions, which may also be aerosolised. Skin lesions are the primary source of transmissible varicella-zoster virus. It is important to note that transmission of varicella-zoster virus typically leads to varicella (chickenpox) in individuals who have not been previously exposed to the virus, rather than herpes zoster (shingles). Varicella-zoster virus has no seasonal variation and occurs throughout the year.

A person with herpes zoster becomes contagious when the rash appears and remains so until the lesions have crusted over. The risk of transmission is lower if the lesions are adequately covered. Herpes zoster is approximately one-fifth as contagious as varicella.

EPIDEMIOLOGY

Herpes zoster occurs worldwide. The incidence (and severity) of shingles increases with age. The overall annual incidence in the UK is estimated to be 1.85–3.9 cases per 1000 population, increasing with age from less than two cases per 1000 in people younger than 50 years to 11 cases per 1000 in people aged 80 years or older (Le 2019). In those people aged 70–79 years, the annual incidence in England and Wales is around 790–880 cases per 100 000 people. The lifetime risk of developing shingles is 20–30% and the risk increases with age (Zorzoli, Pica, and Masetti 2018).

RISK FACTORS

There are a number of risk factors for shingles. Increasing age, although shingles can occur at any age, the incidence of the disease (and the risk of complications) increases with age. This is thought to result from an age-related decline in virus-specific, cell-mediated immune responses.

Immunocompromise and other conditions that change cell-mediated immunity can increase the risk of shingles (and its associated complications). These conditions include HIV infection, lymphoproliferative malignancies, immunosuppressive treatment (such as long-term corticosteroid use and chemotherapy) and organ transplantation. Certain comorbidities, including:

- Rheumatoid arthritis

- Asthma and chronic obstructive pulmonary disease

- Chronic kidney disease

- Depression

- Diabetes

- Systemic lupus erythematosus

- Granulomatosis with polyangiitis, previously known as Wegener's granulomatosis

- Malignancies

Shingles has been linked to physical, emotional and sexual abuse. Other contributing factors may include financial stress, inability to work, decreased independence and an inadequate social support environment.

There is some evidence that women have a greater risk of developing shingles than men. Race/ethnicity, a systematic review and meta-analysis determined that Black people had almost half the risk of shingles as White people (Kawai and Yawn 2017).

In addition to increasing age and having a weakened immune system, there are other risk factors that can lead to complications from shingles.

- Increasing age: Older adults are at higher risk for shingles complications.

- Immunocompromise: People with weakened immune systems (due to illnesses, medications) are also at higher risk.

- Additional risk factors:

  - Severe atopic dermatitis/eczema: People with severe skin conditions such as atopic dermatitis or eczema are more likely to have complications from shingles.

  - Herpes zoster of the head and/or neck area: Shingles affecting the head or neck are more likely to cause serious complications.

Table 7.3 Risk factors associated with herpes zoster

Risk factor	Discussion
Age	The risk increases with age, particularly in people older than 50 years.
Immunosuppression	Conditions such as HIV, cancer or treatments such as chemotherapy can weaken the immune system and increase the risk.
Intrauterine exposure to varicella-zoster virus	Individuals exposed to the varicella-zoster virus in utero may have an increased risk.
Early age of varicella infection	Having chickenpox at younger than 18 months can be a risk factor.
Chronic conditions	Diseases that include asthma and chronic obstructive pulmonary disease may also increase the risk.

Source: Adapted from Leung, Harrington, and Dooling (2021).

- Herpes zoster with specific symptoms: Moderate-to-severe prodromal or acute zoster-associated pain. Significant pain before (prodromal) or during the shingles outbreak indicates a higher risk for complications.

- Severe rash and/or signs of cutaneous dissemination: A widespread rash or signs that the virus has spread across the skin (cutaneous dissemination) suggest a more severe infection.

- Signs of central nervous system involvement: Symptoms that indicate the virus is affecting the brain or spinal cord (e.g. confusion, headaches, difficulty with movement) are serious.

- Signs of visceral involvement: Symptoms that indicate the virus has affected internal organs (visceral involvement), such as difficulty breathing or abdominal pain, are also serious.

Table 7.3 summarises the risk factors associated with herpes zoster.

CLINICAL PRESENTATION

The rash associated with herpes zoster can occur in any dermatome. It most commonly appears on the trunk along the thoracic dermatome or on the face. Dermatomes are specific areas of the skin that are supplied by particular spinal nerves. When herpes zoster reactivates, it typically manifests as a painful rash that follows a specific dermatome pattern. In the case of the trunk, it often appears as a band-like rash that wraps around one side of the torso. This follows the path of the thoracic dermatome, which is supplied by spinal nerves originating from the thoracic (chest) region of the spine.

The varicella-zoster virus typically progresses through distinct phases:

- Pre-eruptive phase (prodromal phase)

Before the rash appears, there is a pre-eruptive phase. During this phase, individuals may experience heightened sensitivity or pain in the affected area. Generalised symptoms include feeling unwell, headache and fever, burning or tingling sensations.

- Eruptive phase

Following the pre-eruptive phase, the eruptive phase begins. In this phase, a rash characterised by fluid-filled blisters develops. The rash typically appears unilaterally (on one side of the body), following a dermatomal distribution (along a specific nerve pathway). The blisters can be painful and may cause itching. Over the course of three to four weeks, the blisters will gradually crust over and heal.

- Post-eruptive phase

After the rash has cleared, some individuals may experience lingering pain in the affected area. This is known as postherpetic neuralgia.

Understanding the progression of varicella-zoster virus and the phases it progresses through can help in recognising and managing symptoms effectively.

A period of hypersensitivity precedes an outbreak of shingles, with complaints of feeling under the weather, headache, fever, burning and pain; this is called the pre-eruptive phase. In the eruptive phase, blisters develop in a unilateral area and take three to four weeks to clear.

Another common location for herpes zoster is on the face. When it affects the face, it typically follows the distribution of the trigeminal nerve, which supplies sensation to the face and forehead. The rash can appear around the eye (known as herpes zoster ophthalmicus), on the forehead or other areas of the face served by branches of the trigeminal nerve.

Those people with weakened immune systems are more likely to have atypical presentations. Postherpetic neuralgia is the most common complication of herpes zoster. This condition affects 30% of people after an episode of shingles. Treatment of people with postherpetic neuralgia is complex, with varying degrees of success in controlling the chronic pain (see Table 7.4).

Table 7.4   Postherpetic neuralgia

Opioid analgesics (narcotics)	Purpose: Provides pain relief for severe or refractory postherpetic neuralgia pain.
	Examples:
	Oxycodone: used for moderate-to-severe pain.
	Morphine: used for severe pain.
	Hydrocodone: often combined with paracetamol for pain relief.
	Administration: taken orally as tablets, capsules or liquids; sometimes available as patches (fentanyl).
	Considerations: side effects such as constipation, nausea and sedation.
Tricyclic antidepressants	Purpose: used for their analgesic properties in neuropathic pain, including postherpetic neuralgia pain.
	Examples:
	Amitriptyline: commonly prescribed for postherpetic neuralgia pain.
	Nortriptyline: has fewer side effects compared to amitriptyline.
	Administration: taken orally in tablet or capsule form.
	Considerations: side effects include dry mouth, constipation, urinary retention and sedation. Tricyclic antidepressants may take several weeks to show full effects.

(Continued)

Table 7.4 (*Continued*)

Anticonvulsants	Purpose: effective for neuropathic pain by stabilising nerve activity.
	Examples:
	Gabapentin: widely used for postherpetic neuralgia pain management.
	Pregabalin: similar to gabapentin but with a more predictable absorption and dosing schedule.
	Administration: taken orally as tablets or capsules.
	Considerations: side effects include dizziness, drowsiness and peripheral oedema. Dosage adjustments may be necessary based on kidney function.
Topical agents	Purpose: provide localised pain relief with fewer systemic side effects.
	Examples:
	Capsaicin cream: derived from chilli peppers; depletes substance P from nerve endings.
	Lidocaine patches: provide localised numbing effect to reduce pain.
	Administration: applied directly to the affected skin area.
	Considerations: capsaicin can cause a burning sensation initially; lidocaine patches should be applied to intact skin and used as directed to avoid systemic absorption.
Transcutaneous electrical nerve stimulation	Purpose: non-pharmacological method to reduce pain through electrical stimulation.
	Mechanism: transcutaneous electrical nerve stimulation units deliver mild electrical pulses to the skin, which may interrupt pain signals and stimulate the release of endorphins.
	Usage: small electrodes are placed on the skin near the painful area and the device is used according to the prescribed schedule.
	Considerations: transcutaneous electrical nerve stimulation is generally safe but should be used under the guidance of a healthcare professional, especially in patients with pacemakers or other implanted devices.
Additional treatments	Non-narcotic analgesics:
	Non-steroidal anti-inflammatory drugs: ibuprofen, naproxen for mild-to-moderate pain.
	Paracetamol: for mild pain relief.
	Corticosteroids: sometimes used to reduce inflammation and acute pain in the early stages of shingles, but not typically for chronic postherpetic neuralgia pain.
	Comprehensive pain management multimodal approach: Combining medications, topical treatments and non-pharmacological therapies to optimise pain control and minimise side effects.
	Psychological support: cognitive-behavioural therapy, relaxation techniques and counselling to help cope with chronic pain.

Source: Adapted from Peters (2019), Leung, Harrington, and Dooling (2021) and Stephens (2022).

Treatment plans should be tailored to the individual patient's pain severity, medical history and response to previous treatments. The patient should be followed up regularly to monitor for efficacy and side effects of treatment and to adjust the treatment regimen as necessary.

Offering people information about the nature of postherpetic neuralgia, potential treatment options and realistic expectations for pain management can help in the provision of high-quality effective care. The management of postherpetic neuralgia often requires a multidisciplinary approach, incorporating both pharmacological and non-pharmacological strategies to achieve optimal pain relief and improve quality of life.

CLINICAL INVESTIGATIONS AND DIAGNOSIS

The signs and symptoms of herpes zoster are usually distinctive enough to make an accurate clinical diagnosis once the rash appears, but in atypical cases, investigations such as herpes serology are necessary. A history and physical examination are required.

MEDICAL HISTORY

The patient is asked about their symptoms, including the nature of the rash, when it started and any preceding pain or tingling sensations. They will also be asked about their medical history, including any history of chickenpox (since herpes zoster is caused by the reactivation of the varicella-zoster virus, which causes chickenpox).

PHYSICAL EXAMINATION

The characteristic rash associated with herpes zoster is usually sufficient for diagnosis. It typically involves assessing the characteristic skin rash and other related symptoms. Informed consent must be gained, a chaperone offered and adherence to local infection prevention and control policies and procedures.

Visual Inspection of the Skin Rash The patient is observed for a unilateral, dermatomal distribution of the rash. Herpes zoster commonly affects thoracic dermatomes but can also occur on the face, neck or other body parts. The rash does not cross the midline.

The rash usually starts as erythematous (red) macules and papules that progress to grouped vesicles (blisters) on an erythematous base. Over time, these vesicles can become pustular and then crust over.

The presence of lesions in various stages of development (new vesicles, pustules, crusts) can help confirm the diagnosis.

Assessment of Pain and Sensation Patients often report significant pain, burning or tingling in the affected dermatome before the rash appears. The severity and nature of this pain is assessed. The affected area may be hypersensitive (hyperaesthesia) or have reduced sensation (hypoaesthesia). Sensory testing may be performed to evaluate these changes.

Examination of Surrounding Skin The surrounding skin may show signs of inflammation and oedema (swelling). Examination is undertaken for signs of secondary bacterial infection in the lesions, such as increased redness, warmth or purulent discharge.

Inspection of Other Body Parts In cases of herpes zoster affecting the trigeminal nerve, the patient is examined for lesions inside the mouth. The eyes are examined if the ophthalmic branch of the trigeminal nerve is involved (herpes zoster ophthalmicus). Checks are undertaken for eye involvement, including conjunctivitis, keratitis or uveitis. The patient is examined for vesicles in the ear canal and checks for facial nerve palsy.

Lymph Node Examination The lymph nodes are palpated for an enlargement near the affected dermatome, which can occur due to the viral infection. During the physical examination, it is also important to differentiate herpes zoster from other conditions with similar presentations, such as:

- HSV infection: typically involves grouped vesicles but often recurs in the same location and does not follow a dermatomal distribution.

- Contact dermatitis: can cause a rash and itching but usually lacks the preceding pain and follows exposure to an allergen or irritant.

- Impetigo: a bacterial infection that can cause pustular lesions, but these are usually more superficial and widespread without a dermatomal pattern.

The findings of the physical examination should be meticulously documented, including the description of the rash, its distribution and the presence of any complications.

To diagnose atypical presentations of viral infections, electron microscopy of blister fluid, viral culture from swab and skin biopsy are essential (see Table 7.5).

Table 7.5 Overview of investigations that may be used in the diagnosis of herpes zoster

Investigation	Discussion
Viral culture	This process entails cultivating the virus from a sample extracted from the rash or blister fluid. It confirms the existence of the varicella-zoster virus and aids in identifying its specific strain.
Blood tests	This involves testing for antibodies that are produced by the immune system in response to varicella-zoster virus infection. It has the potential to indicate past or current infection.
Electron microscopy	This technique allows for the visualisation of viral particles. This is less commonly used today due to advances in molecular techniques; however, it can still be employed in some cases.
Smear	A sample of fluid from the rash or blister is examined under a microscope for the presence of varicella-zoster virus.
HIV status checking	In specific situations, it is crucial to evaluate HIV status because HIV can compromise the immune system, increasing susceptibility to infections such as herpes zoster.
Polymerase chain reaction testing	A highly sensitive molecular technique used to detect viral DNA in samples. It can provide rapid and accurate results, particularly useful in urgent situations or when a speedy diagnosis is needed.

Source: Adapted from Chowdhury, Katugampola, and Finlay (2019).

These investigations help in confirming the diagnosis of herpes zoster, determining the extent of the infection and guiding appropriate treatment. A comprehensive approach that includes a detailed medical history, thorough physical examination and appropriate investigations is critical in the management of herpes zoster. It ensures accurate diagnosis, identifies potential complications, guides effective treatment, advises patients and addresses public health concerns. This holistic approach ultimately improves patient outcomes and helps prevent the spread of the virus.

MANAGEMENT

Managing herpes zoster involves a combination of antiviral therapy, pain management and supportive care to alleviate symptoms and prevent complications.

ANTIVIRAL THERAPY

Antiviral medications are most effective when started within 72 hours of rash onset. These drugs can reduce the severity and duration of symptoms, as well as the risk of complications. Antiviral medications can be administered both orally and topically, depending on the type of infection and the specific medication (Chowdhury, Katugampola, and Finlay 2019; Stephens 2022).

PAIN MANAGEMENT

Pain associated with shingles can be significant and managing it is a crucial aspect of treatment. In acute pain, non-steroidal anti-inflammatory drugs (NSAIDs) are used. For pain relief, paracetamol can be given. For severe pain, opioids may be prescribed. Topical agents such as lidocaine patches or capsaicin cream may be used.

See Table 7.4 with regard to postherpetic neuralgia.

SUPPORTIVE CARE

Keeping the rash clean and dry to prevent secondary bacterial infection is important.

The patient should be encouraged to stay hydrated and rest. Stephens (2022) suggests that loose-fitting cotton clothing can reduce the risk of irritation.

MANAGEMENT OF COMPLICATIONS

If the rash becomes infected, antibiotics may be required. Herpes zoster ophthalmicus requires urgent ophthalmological consultation and treatment to prevent vision loss.

Rare complications such as meningitis, encephalitis or motor neuropathy need specialist care.

While herpes zoster itself is not contagious, the varicella-zoster virus can be transmitted to individuals who have not had chickenpox or the vaccine, causing chickenpox. Patients should cover the rash and practice good hygiene.

PSYCHOLOGICAL SUPPORT

Chronic pain and discomfort can lead to emotional distress, so providing psychological support or counselling might be necessary.

The effective management of herpes zoster requires a holistic approach tailored to the individual patient's needs, focusing on early antiviral treatment, pain management and preventing complications through vigilant care and patient education.

HEALTH TEACHING

Health teaching for patients with herpes zoster is crucial to help manage the condition effectively and minimise complications. Key aspects of health teaching needs are noted in Table 7.6.

Table 7.6   Key aspects of health teaching needs for people with herpes zoster

Component	Discussion
Understanding herpes zoster	Explain that herpes zoster is caused by the reactivation of the varicella-zoster virus, the same virus that causes chickenpox.
	Clarify that anyone who has had chickenpox can develop shingles, as the virus remains dormant in nerve tissue and can reactivate later in life.
Symptoms and progression	Offer patients information and advice about the typical symptoms of shingles, including a painful rash that usually appears on one side of the body, along with tingling, burning or itching sensations.
	Discuss how the rash evolves from red patches to fluid-filled blisters, which then crust over and heal over several weeks.
Transmission	Emphasise that shingles itself is not contagious, but the varicella-zoster virus can be transmitted to individuals who have not had chickenpox or the chickenpox vaccine, potentially causing chickenpox rather than shingles.
Treatment options	Outline treatment options such as antiviral medications to reduce the severity and duration of the illness.
	Discuss the importance of starting treatment as early as possible, ideally within 72 hours of rash onset, to maximise effectiveness.
Pain management	Address pain management strategies, including over-the-counter pain relievers and prescription medications if necessary.
	Provide guidance on topical treatments or creams that may help alleviate discomfort.
Complications and risks	Offer information and advice about potential complications of shingles, such as postherpetic neuralgia (persistent nerve pain after rash healing), which can be debilitating and long-lasting.
	Discuss other less common but serious complications such as bacterial skin infections.
Self-care and prevention	Advise on self-care measures to promote healing, such as keeping the rash clean and dry, avoiding scratching and using cool compresses to soothe the skin.
	Encourage patients to rest and avoid strenuous activities that could exacerbate symptoms.

Component	Discussion
Vaccination	Recommend the importance of vaccination against shingles, even if the person has had shingles previously.
	Explain the benefits of vaccination in reducing the risk of developing shingles and its complications.
Follow-up and monitoring	Stress the need for follow-up appointments with healthcare providers to monitor healing progress, manage symptoms and address any concerns or new symptoms promptly.
Psychosocial support	Acknowledge the emotional impact of shingles, especially if it causes discomfort, disruption of daily activities or anxiety about potential complications.
	Offer resources or referrals to support groups, if available, where patients can connect with others experiencing similar challenges.

Providing comprehensive health teaching on these topics, those who offer care and support can empower patients with herpes zoster to actively participate in their care, promote faster recovery and prevent future occurrences or complications.

VACCINATION

A shingles vaccination programme was introduced in September 2013 in the UK. A national shingles immunisation programme was introduced for adults aged 70 years. A phased catch-up programme was included for adults aged 71–79 years. The vaccine used was a single dose of a live, attenuated virus vaccine. The decision to target the 70–79 years age group was based on evidence showing the cost-effectiveness of vaccinating this group. Reasons for targeting this age group include:

- Burden of shingles: Shingles incidence and severity increase with age, making older adults more vulnerable.

- Vaccine effectiveness: The vaccine's efficacy decreases with age, so it is more effective when given at a younger age within this group.

- Duration of protection: The vaccine provides sufficient immunity for individuals in this age group, offering protection for a significant period following vaccination.

Adults should receive two doses of the vaccine a minimum of eight weeks apart (UKHSA 2024).

The vaccine should be given via intramuscular injection, preferably in the deltoid region of the upper arm. Subcutaneous administration is not advised. Caution is necessary when administering the vaccine to individuals with thrombocytopenia or any coagulation disorder, as there is a risk of bleeding following intramuscular administration. The vaccine should never be given intravascularly.

When the vaccine is administered concurrently with another vaccine, they should be given at separate injection sites, preferably in different limbs. If administered in the same limb, they should be spaced at least 2.5 cm apart. The vaccine should not be given to individuals with a history of a confirmed anaphylactic reaction to any component of the vaccine (UKHSA 2024).

The most commonly reported side effects associated with the vaccine include:

- Pain at the injection site (68%)

- Myalgia (muscle pain) (33%)

- Fatigue (32%)

These reactions are typically short-lived, with a median duration of two to three days.

The site at which each vaccine was given should be noted in the individual's record/ notes.

Revisions to age groups eligible for the vaccine are being made.

CONCLUSION

Understanding herpes zoster (shingles) is essential in order to offer effective care and education to patients. This chapter has explored the pathophysiology, clinical manifestations, treatment options and preventive measures associated with this viral infection. Herpes zoster can significantly impact patients' quality of life due to its painful symptoms and potential complications, such as postherpetic neuralgia.

By promoting vaccination and providing comprehensive health teaching on symptom management, pain relief strategies and infection control measures, those who offer care and support can empower patients to actively participate in their recovery and minimise the risk of recurrent episodes.

Adopting empathy and understanding for the physical and emotional toll of herpes zoster on patients is paramount. By integrating holistic care principles into practice, we can support patients through their journey with herpes zoster, promoting comfort, healing and improved outcomes.

GLOSSARY OF TERMS

Acute: Refers to the initial phase of herpes zoster when symptoms such as pain and rash are actively present.

Antiviral medications: Medications such as acyclovir, valacyclovir and famciclovir used to treat herpes zoster by inhibiting viral replication.

Complications: Potential adverse outcomes associated with herpes zoster, including postherpetic neuralgia, bacterial infections of the skin and ocular complications.

Dermatome: Area of skin supplied by a single spinal nerve. Herpes zoster typically affects a specific dermatome.

Differential diagnosis: Process of distinguishing herpes zoster from other conditions with similar symptoms, such as herpes simplex virus, dermatitis or cellulitis.

Herpes zoster: Viral infection caused by reactivation of the varicella-zoster virus, characterised by a painful rash with fluid-filled blisters on one side of the body.

Herpes zoster ophthalmicus: Herpes zoster affecting the ophthalmic division of the trigeminal nerve, potentially leading to eye complications.

Immunisation: Process of inducing immunity against herpes zoster through vaccination, reducing the risk and severity of the disease.

Immunocompromised: Having a weakened immune system, which can increase the risk and severity of herpes zoster.

Postherpetic neuralgia: Persistent nerve pain following resolution of the herpes zoster rash, lasting for months to years in some cases.

Prodrome: Early symptoms that precede the onset of the herpes zoster rash, including pain, tingling or itching in the affected dermatome.

Reactivation: Awakening of the dormant varicella-zoster virus in nerve cells, leading to the development of herpes zoster.

Varicella-zoster virus: Virus responsible for both chickenpox (primary infection) and herpes zoster (reactivation infection).

Vesicles: Small, fluid-filled blisters that appear on the skin during the active phase of herpes zoster.

Vesicular rash: Rash characterised by fluid-filled blisters (vesicles), a hallmark of the herpes zoster rash.

MULTIPLE CHOICE QUESTIONS

1. What virus causes herpes zoster?
   a) Herpes simplex virus
   b) Varicella-zoster virus
   c) Epstein–Barr virus
   d) Cytomegalovirus

2. What is the common name for herpes zoster?
   a) Cold sores
   b) Genital herpes
   c) Shingles
   d) Chickenpox

3. Which age group is most commonly affected by herpes zoster?
   a) Children under 12 years
   b) Adolescents
   c) Adults over 50 years
   d) Young adults

4. What is the recommended site for intramuscular administration of the vaccine?
   a) Gluteus maximus
   b) Deltoid region of the upper arm
   c) Thigh
   d) Abdomen

5. Which of the following is a common complication of herpes zoster?
   a) Postherpetic neuralgia
   b) Meningitis
   c) Encephalitis
   d) Pneumonia

6. What is the first-line antiviral treatment for herpes zoster?
   a) Amoxicillin
   b) Acyclovir
   c) Azithromycin
   d) Ibuprofen

7. Herpes zoster typically presents with a rash that is:
   a) Bilateral and symmetrical
   b) Unilateral and follows a dermatome
   c) Spread all over the body
   d) Limited to the face

8. What is a common early symptom (prodrome) of herpes zoster?
   a) Fever and chills
   b) Pain and tingling in the affected area
   c) Cough and sore throat
   d) Diarrhoea

9. Which complication of herpes zoster affects the eye?
   a) Herpes zoster oticus
   b) Herpes zoster ophthalmicus
   c) Herpes zoster sinusitis
   d) Herpes zoster dermatitis

10. Which of the following is NOT recommended for managing pain in herpes zoster?
    a) Antiviral medications
    b) Topical anaesthetics
    c) Acetaminophen
    d) Subcutaneous injection of steroids

REFERENCES

Chowdhury, M.M., Katugampola, R.P., and Finlay, A.Y. (2019). *Dermatology at a Glance*, 2e. Oxford: Wiley.

Kawai, K. and Yawn, B.P. (2017). Risk factors for herpes zoster: a systematic review and meta-analysis. *Mayo Clinic Proceedings* 92 (12): 1806–1821. https://www.mayoclinicproceedings.org/article/S0025-6196(17)30742-5/abstract.

Le, P. (2019). Herpes zoster infection. *British Medical Journal* 364. https://www.bmj.com/content/364/bmj.k5095.

Leung, J., Harrington, T., and Dooling, K. (2021). Zoster. Pinkbook: Herpes zoster. https://www.cdc.gov/pinkbook/hcp/table-of-contents/chapter-23-zoster.html (accessed June 2024).

Peters, J. (2019). Nursing patients with skin disorders (Chapter 13). In: *Alexander's Nursing Practice*, 5e (ed. I. Peate). London: Elsevier.

Steinmann, M., Lampe, D., Grosser, J. (2023). Risk factors for herpes zoster infections: a systematic review and meta-analysis unveiling common trends and heterogeneity patterns. *Infection* 52 (3): 1009–1026. https://pubmed.ncbi.nlm.nih.gov/38236326/.

Stephens, M. (2022). The person with a skin disorder (Chapter 35). In: *Nursing Practice*, 3e (ed. I. Peate and Mitchell). Oxford: Wiley.

UK Health Security Agency (2024). Shingles (herpes zoster): the green book (Chapter 28). https://assets.publishing.service.gov.uk/media/6603fedef9ab41001aeea371/Shingles_Green_Book_chapter_28a_20240315.pdf (accessed 2024).

Zorzoli, E., Pica, F., Masetti, G. (2018). Herpes zoster in frail elderly patients: prevalence, impact, management, and preventive strategies. *Aging Clinical and Experimental Research* 30 (7): 693–702. https://pubmed.ncbi.nlm.nih.gov/29721782/.

Acne Vulgaris CHAPTER 8

ACNE

Acne is a disorder of the pilosebaceous apparatus characterised by comedones, papules, pustules, cysts and scars (Weller, Hunter, and Mann 2014). This is a general term that encompasses a number of skin conditions that can occur in various forms and severities.

Many patients with skin diseases experience a significant impact on their quality of life, though some manage to continue their lives as usual (see Figure 8.1). Chronic inflammatory skin conditions, such as severe psoriasis, eczema and acne, often cause the most substantial impairments to quality of life. Additionally, disfiguring diseases, for example, vitiligo and alopecia areata, can lead to serious issues (Peate 2019). Virtually all aspects of patients' lives can be affected, including home care, shopping, clothing choices, social activities, sports, study, work and personal and sexual relationships. Patients often experience itchiness and embarrassment and the treatments, particularly topical ones, can further add to their burden.

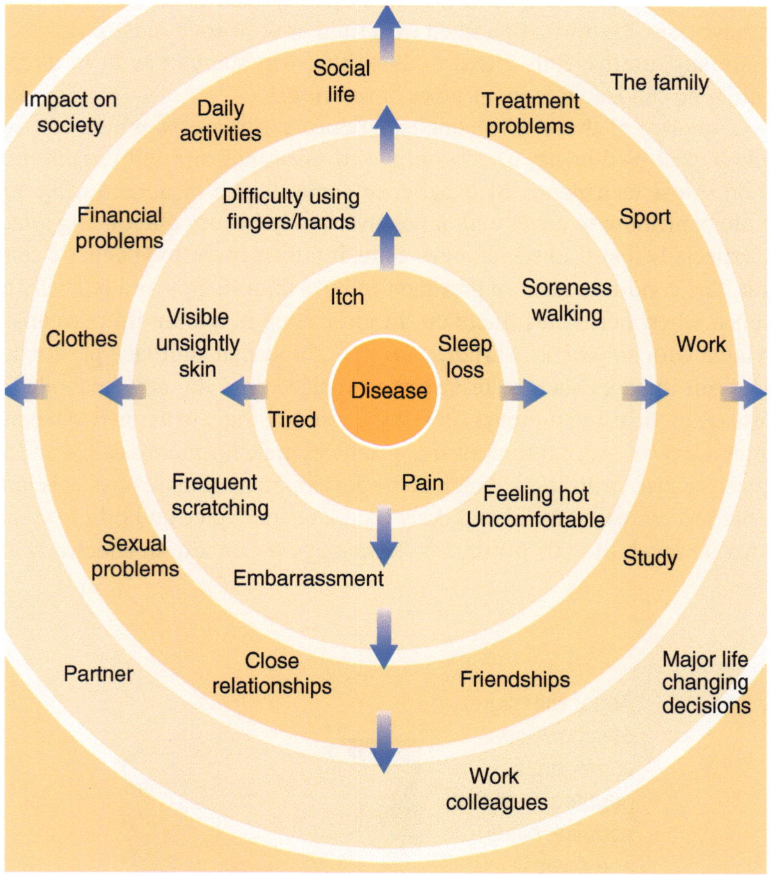

FIGURE 8.1   The impact of skin conditions

PATHOPHYSIOLOGICAL CHANGES ASSOCIATED WITH ACNE VULGARIS

Acne vulgaris is a common skin condition that affects most individuals in the UK at some point in their lives. The pathogenesis of acne vulgaris is not completely understood (Primary Care Dermatology Society 2023). Acne vulgaris is defined as a chronic, inflammatory skin disease primarily presenting with open or closed comedones, papules, pustules or nodules on the face or trunk and may result in pain, erythema, hyperpigmentation or scars (American Academy of Dermatology 2024). It is a disorder of the pilosebaceous follicles (Peters 2019). During puberty, androgens increase the production of sebum from enlarged sebaceous glands, leading to blockages and infections with *Propionibacterium acnes* (*P. acnes*), causing an inflammatory reaction. Comedones, which are follicles blocked and distended by partially desquamated keratinocytes and sebum, can be open (blackheads) or closed (whiteheads). Inflammation can further result in papules, pustules and nodules (see Figure 8.2).

Papules are small, erythematous (red) bumps on the skin, measuring 2–5 mm in diameter. They are relatively deep within the skin. Pustules are similar in size to papules (2–5 mm in diameter) but contain pus. They are more superficial than papules. Nodules are larger and deeper than papules; these are solid, inflamed lumps under the skin. Nodules resemble inflamed epidermoid cysts (a type of benign skin cyst) but do not have a true cystic structure (they do not have a sac-like formation filled with fluid or semi-solid material).

Cysts are suppurative (pus-filled) nodules that can sometimes form deep abscesses. Chronic cystic acne can lead to various types of scarring.

Nearly a quarter of those with acne experience severe cases, which can significantly impact psychological well-being, undermining self-assurance and self-esteem during a vulnerable period. Most teenagers will experience some degree of acne during adolescence. Genetic factors contribute to acne, with a positive family history often being a factor. When both twins (especially identical twins) have acne, it indicates a strong genetic component to the condition. The condition is more prevalent in boys than in girls and typically occurs during adolescence when hormones fluctuate. In girls, acne may flare up premenstrually and can be associated with polycystic ovarian syndrome. Abnormal androgen production can also lead to acne, seen in cases such as testosterone replacement therapy, anabolic steroid use, Cushing's disease or virilising tumours such as arrhenoblastoma in women. Arrhenoblastoma is an uncommon type of ovarian tumour that produces male hormones called androgens. The excess androgens cause virilisation, which is the development of male physical characteristics in females, such as increased facial and body hair, a deeper voice and other symptoms associated with higher levels of male hormones. To manage the condition effectively and achieve

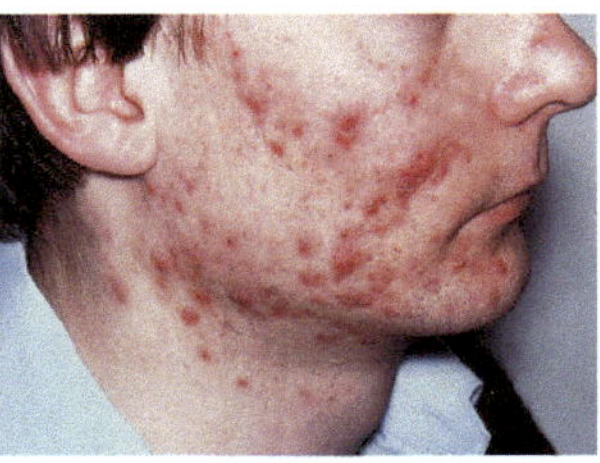

FIGURE 8.2 Acne. *Source:* Davey et al., (2024). With permission from John Wiley & Sons.

the best possible health results, it is important to diagnose the tumour early and remove it, usually surgically.

Acne vulgaris is almost universal in adolescence, with 1% of men and 5% of women requiring treatment up to the age of 40 years. This chronic disorder results in increased sebum production, ductal hypercornification, a disturbed relationship with commensal microorganisms (*P. acnes*) and cutaneous inflammation. Increased sebum production is likely the fundamental abnormality.

Sebaceous glands are driven by androgens and women with acne vulgaris often exhibit a complex form of cutaneous androgenisation. Many women with acne vulgaris have polycystic ovaries detectable via ultrasonography, although most do not exhibit other features of polycystic ovary syndrome. There is no evidence for systemic endocrine abnormalities in men.

The pathogenesis of acne vulgaris is multifactorial (American Academy of Dermatology 2024). The significant factor is genetics. Acne vulgaris develops as a result of an interplay of the following four factors:

1. Follicular epidermal hyperproliferation with subsequent plugging of the follicle

2. Excess sebum production

3. The presence and activity of the commensal bacteria *P. acnes*

4. Inflammation (see Figure 8.3)

(Davey 2024)

Retention hyperkeratosis (the excessive accumulation of skin cells within hair follicles, leading to clogged pores) is the first recognised event in the development of acne vulgaris. The exact cause of this excessive cell proliferation is unknown, but androgen hormones (testosterone) are believed to be a trigger. Comedones, the clinical lesions resulting from follicular plugging, start appearing around puberty (adrenarche) in individuals with acne, particularly in the T-zone area. The severity of comedonal acne in prepubertal girls correlates with circulating levels of the adrenal androgen dehydroepiandrosterone sulphate. Moreover, androgen hormone receptors are present in sebaceous glands and individuals with malfunctioning androgen receptors do not develop acne.

Excess sebum production is another significant factor in the development of acne vulgaris. Sebum production and excretion are regulated by various hormones and mediators.

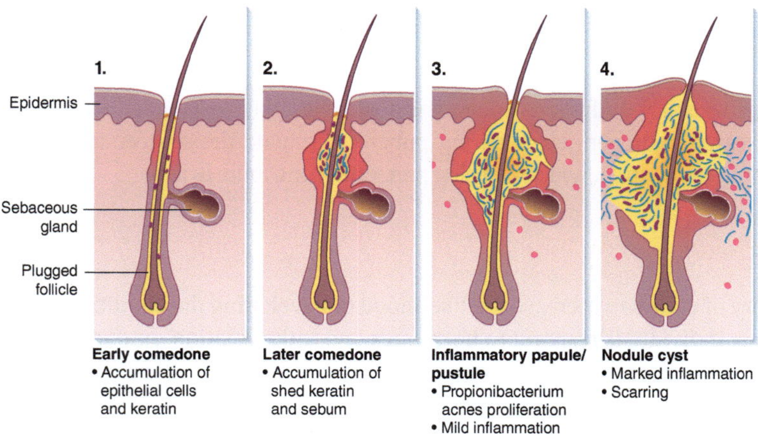

FIGURE 8.3 The pathogenesis of acne vulgaris

Androgen hormones promote sebum production and release, yet most individuals with acne vulgaris have normal circulating levels of androgens. Other regulators, such as growth hormone and insulin-like growth factor, also influence the sebaceous glands and contribute to acne development.

Propionibacterium acnes, an anaerobic organism, is present in acne lesions and promotes inflammation. It stimulates the production of pro-inflammatory mediators that diffuse through the follicle wall. *P. acnes* stimulates monocytes and neutrophils, leading to the production of multiple pro-inflammatory cytokines, including interleukins-12 and -8 and tumour necrosis factor. Hypersensitivity to *P. acnes* may explain why some individuals develop inflammatory acne vulgaris while others do not.

EPIDEMIOLOGY

Approximately 9% of the global population is affected by acne. The prevalence of acne varies significantly across different regions, with Western industrialised countries experiencing much higher rates compared to some non-industrialised nations (American Academy of Dermatology 2024).

In Western industrialised countries, up to 95% of adolescents experience some form of acne, with 20–35% developing moderate to severe cases (Heng and Chew 2020). Among those with acne:

- 85% are aged 12–24 years

- 8% are aged 25–34 years

- 3% are aged 35–44 years

Acne is more prevalent in males during adolescence, but the incidence is higher in women during adulthood. In the UK, acne is one of the most common skin conditions, leading to 3.5 million visits to primary care each year.

RISK FACTORS

Acne vulgaris is influenced by various risk factors that can contribute to its development and severity. Risk factors for acne development include hormonal changes during adolescence, family history of acne and oily skin type (Heng and Chew 2020).

HORMONAL CHANGES

Hormones, particularly androgens such as testosterone, play a significant role in acne development. Increased androgen levels during puberty stimulate the sebaceous glands, leading to excessive sebum production, which can clog pores and contribute to acne.

GENETICS

Family history of acne can increase the likelihood of developing the condition. Genetic factors influence how individuals respond to hormones and inflammation, impacting their susceptibility to acne.

SEBUM PRODUCTION

Excessive sebum production, influenced by hormonal factors, can contribute to acne formation. Individuals with oily skin types are more prone to developing acne due to the increased likelihood of pores becoming clogged.

SKIN CARE PRODUCTS

Certain cosmetics and skin care products, especially those that are oil-based or comedogenic (tend to clog pores), can exacerbate acne by blocking pores and promoting bacterial growth.

DIET

While the direct impact of diet on acne is debated, some studies suggest that high glycaemic index foods and dairy products may worsen acne in susceptible individuals. However, more research is needed to establish clear causal relationships.

STRESS

Psychological stress can exacerbate acne by increasing inflammation and altering hormone levels. Stress management techniques may help reduce acne severity in some individuals.

MEDICATIONS

Certain medications, such as corticosteroids, lithium and some anticonvulsants, can trigger or worsen acne outbreaks by affecting hormone levels or increasing sebum production.

ENVIRONMENTAL FACTORS

Exposure to pollutants, high humidity and sweating can contribute to acne development by clogging pores and promoting bacterial growth on the skin.

MENSTRUAL CYCLE

Hormonal fluctuations during the menstrual cycle can lead to increased sebum production and pore blockage, contributing to acne flare-ups in women.

OCCUPATIONAL FACTORS

Exposure to oils, greases and certain chemicals in certain occupations (e.g. cooking, mechanics) may increase the risk of developing acne due to pore-clogging substances contacting the skin regularly.

Understanding these risk factors helps in identifying potential triggers for acne vulgaris and implementing targeted prevention strategies and treatment approaches. Management of acne vulgaris often involves a multifaceted approach tailored to individual needs, addressing both the underlying causes and the symptoms of the condition.

Table 8.1 Acne vulgaris and acne conglobate

Type of acne	Clinical presentation
Acne vulgaris	Common in teenagers and young to middle-aged adults
	The cause is unknown but a possible androgenic influence on sebaceous glands. The condition can be:
	Mild: a few scattered comedones and occasional papules
	Moderate: presence of comedones, macules, papules and pustules
	Severe: comedones, papules and pustules, painful nodules and cysts resulting in scar formation and causing pigment changes
Acne conglobata	Occurs in middle years
	Cause unknown
	Serious skin lesions occur, with discharge ranging from serous to purulent. Has an offensive odour

Source: Adapted from Stephens (2022).

CLINICAL PRESENTATION

Acne typically appears on parts of the body with a high concentration of pilosebaceous glands, including the face, chest and back. The clinical features of acne can vary greatly based on its severity and the individual affected. For a diagnosis of acne, the presence of comedones is essential; if they are absent, other diagnoses should be explored (Leung et al. 2021; Primary Care Dermatology Society 2023).

The condition is characterised by non-inflammatory lesions, such as open or closed comedones, as well as inflammatory lesions, including papules, pustules and nodules; the affected person typically has oily skin. Local symptoms can include pain or tenderness. There are generally no systemic symptoms in acne vulgaris. However, severe acne with systemic signs and symptoms, such as fever, is known as acne fulminans. This acute, severe form of acne presents with fever, joint pain (arthralgia) and non-infectious bone lesions (Davey 2024). Severe acne with multiple comedones but without systemic symptoms is referred to as acne conglobata. This severe type of acne often leads to disfiguring scars.

See Table 8.1 for an overview of acne vulgaris and acne conglobata.

CLINICAL INVESTIGATIONS AND DIAGNOSIS

Making a diagnosis of acne vulgaris usually includes a comprehensive medical history and a detailed physical examination. Other clinical investigations may be required.

MEDICAL HISTORY

The following are discussed when gathering a medical history:

- Onset and duration: determining when the acne started and how long it has been present. The patient is asked about the distribution of lesions.

- Progression: understanding how the acne has evolved over time, including any changes in severity. Determine if there are any exacerbating factors, for example, flares with menstruation, contraceptives, use of cosmetics, face creams or hair pomades.

- Past treatments: reviewing any previous treatments or medications used for acne, including over-the-counter and prescription products and their effectiveness.

- Medications: identifying any medications currently being taken that could potentially cause or worsen acne, such as corticosteroids, lithium or certain oral contraceptives.

- Family history: checking for any family history of acne or related dermatological conditions.

The psychosocial impact of acne can be profound, affecting various aspects of an individual's life. During the clinical evaluation, it is important to assess the psychological and social repercussions of acne. Table 8.2 discusses the psychological and social assessment, the impact of acne and history taking.

Table 8.2   History taking – the psychological and social impact of acne

Psychological and social impact	Discussion
Psychological assessment:	
Emotional well-being	Sensitive inquiries are asked about the patient's general emotional state. Questions can include:
	'How do you feel about your skin condition?'
	'Do you find that your acne affects your mood or self-esteem?'
Anxiety and depression	There may be a need to screen the patient for symptoms of anxiety and depression, which are common among patients with acne. Validated screening tools such as the Generalised Anxiety Disorder 7-item (GAD-7) scale or the Patient Health Questionnaire-9 (PHQ-9) may be used.
	The patient is asked direct questions such as:
	'Do you feel anxious or worried about your acne or its impact on your life?'
	'Have you experienced feelings of sadness, hopelessness or a loss of interest in activities you used to enjoy?'
Social impact:	
Interpersonal relationships	Tactfully, explorations are made with how acne can affect the patient's relationships with family, friends and peers. Questions can include:
	'Do you find it difficult to interact with others because of your acne?'
	'Has acne affected your social life or activities you participate in?'
Social avoidance	It is determined if the patient avoids social situations due to embarrassment or self-consciousness about their skin. Ask:
	'Have you ever avoided going out or attending events because of your acne?'
	'Do you feel self-conscious in social settings due to your skin condition?'

(Continued)

Table 8.2 (*Continued*)

Psychological and social impact	Discussion
Impact on daily activities:	
School or work performance	Assess whether acne affects the patient's performance or participation in school or work. Questions might include:
	'Has your acne affected your concentration or performance at school/work?'
	'Do you feel that your acne has impacted your professional opportunities or ambitions?'
Daily routine	Understand how acne influences the patient's daily routines, including grooming and skincare habits:
	'Do you spend a lot of time trying to manage or cover up your acne?'
	'Has your skincare routine or the need to manage your acne disrupted your daily life?'
Body image and self-esteem	Self-perception: Explore how acne impacts the patient's body image and self-esteem. Questions can include:
	'How do you feel about your appearance when you look in the mirror?'
	'Do you feel less confident because of your acne?'
	Comparison to others: Investigate if the patient frequently compares their skin to others, which can negatively affect self-esteem:
	'Do you often compare your skin to others' and feel bad about it?'
	'Do you feel pressure to have clear skin because of social media or societal standards?'
Coping mechanisms and support systems:	
Coping strategies	The patient is asked about how they cope with the emotional and social challenges of acne:
	'How do you manage the emotional impact of your acne?'
	'Are there any strategies or activities that help you feel better about your skin?'
	Support network: Determine the availability and quality of the patient's support network, including family, friends and support groups:
	'Do you have friends or family members you can talk to about your acne?'
	'Have you ever joined a support group or online community for people with acne?'

If significant psychological distress is identified, consideration is given to referring the patient to a mental health professional for further evaluation and support.

Thoroughly exploring these areas can provide a comprehensive understanding of the psychosocial impact of acne on the patient and offers holistic, empathetic care that addresses both physical and emotional needs.

PHYSICAL EXAMINATION

A physical examination is essential in making a diagnosis of acne and in determining the extent of lesions. Local policy and procedure must be adhered to with regards to consent, infection prevention and control and the provision of a chaperone. Vital signs are taken and recorded. The patient is observed for:

- Type and distribution of lesions: evaluating the types of lesions present (comedones, papules, pustules, nodules, cysts) and their locations on the body (face, chest, back, shoulders).

- Severity assessment: classifying the acne severity (mild, moderate, severe) based on the number and types of lesions.

- Presence of scarring: noting any scarring or post-inflammatory hyperpigmentation, which may indicate chronic or severe acne.

- Skin type: assessing the patient's skin type (oily, dry, combination), which can influence the choice of treatment.

INVESTIGATIONS

There are usually no investigations required to make a diagnosis. Occasionally, if investigations are required, this is to explore a possible underlying cause, such as a virilising tumour. Skin lesion culture may be necessary in those who do not respond to treatment. This is to exclude Gram-negative folliculitis.

MANAGEMENT

The condition typically resolves on its own over time. Treatment varies based on severity, and maintaining an objective record of it aids in monitoring progress. Using photographs can help track development of the condition. Treatment focuses on keeping the skin clean, preventing microbial growth and using keratolytics (they work by breaking down the bonds between dead skin cells, which can clog pores that contribute to acne) to alleviate comedones. Care provision requires a full assessment of the severity of the acne (Stephens 2022).

The face should be kept clean with twice-daily washing using soap and water, not more than twice per day (Primary Care Dermatology Society 2023). Branded antiseptic products may be beneficial. Laser treatment with a 1450 nm laser can improve acne. This is a specific type of laser that targets and heats the sebaceous glands in the skin. By doing so, it reduces the production of sebum (skin oil) and can also diminish inflammation associated with acne. This treatment is typically used for individuals with moderate-to-severe acne who have not responded well to other conventional treatments such as topical medications or oral antibiotics (American Academy of Dermatology 2024). The laser treatment aims to achieve clearer skin by addressing the underlying causes of acne, such as excess sebum production and inflammation. Blue light phototherapy (a non-invasive and effective treatment option for inflammatory acne, targeting *P. acnes* bacteria to reduce inflammation and promote clearer skin) is effective for mild-to-moderate papulopustular acne. Topical treatments should cover all affected areas, not just existing lesions. Salicylic acid 10% works similarly to retinoids. Benzoyl peroxide reduces sebum production

Table 8.3 Treatment overview

Severity	Treatment
Mild acne	Topical antibiotics, keratolytics and retinoids.
Moderate-to-severe acne	There may be a need for both topical and systemic therapy, with oral antibiotics (which can result in failure of the oral contraceptive pill or teratogenicity) or antiandrogenic hormones (i.e. for women, a suitable contraceptive pill).
Severe nodulocystic (conglobate) acne or failure to respond to other treatments	There is an indication for the oral retinoid (vitamin A derivative) isotretinoin (13-cis-retinoic acid). This highly effective drug affects all four aetiological factors operating in acne and reduces sebum production by 75–90%. Treatment lasts six to eight months. Side effects, which are essentially those of hypervitaminosis A, include teratogenesis (women must not get pregnant when on treatment), eczema, cheilitis (sore lips), conjunctivitis, benign intracranial hypertension, mood disturbance and biochemical hepatitis and hyperlipidaemia.

Source: Adapted from Davey (2024).

and comedones and inhibits *P. acnes* growth for mild papulopustular acne. Topical antibiotics such as erythromycin, clindamycin and tetracycline can also be effective. Local treatment with topical retinoids such as isotretinoin, tretinoin or adapalene reduces comedones and has anti-inflammatory effects. Systemic treatments may take several months to show improvement and should be continued for three to four months if tolerated, often in combination with topical treatments. No oral antibiotic has been shown to be consistently superior in terms of effectiveness, tolerability or safety. Anti-androgen treatments, particularly oestrogenic oral contraceptives, are effective for acne. Laser resurfacing, dermabrasion and chemical peels are used to treat scarring. Microdermabrasion is a straightforward outpatient procedure involving blowing abrasive substances such as aluminium oxide crystals onto the face and vacuuming them off. Dermabrasion, mechanical dermabrasion and ablative laser treatment of the entire face or non-facial regions are not recommended within six months of isotretinoin use due to increased risks of adverse events (Waldman et al. 2017). Table 8.3 provides an overview of treatment regimens.

Most treatments do not change the natural course of the condition, with the exception of isotretinoin. Isotretinoin is a retinoid, derived from vitamin A, and works by reducing the amount of oil released by oil glands in the skin, promoting skin cell turnover and decreasing inflammation.

LONG-TERM TREATMENT REQUIREMENT

Topical therapies are necessary over an extended period to manage acne effectively. They help control symptoms and prevent new outbreaks. Antibiotics should be used for at least six months to effectively reduce acne-causing bacteria. Sometimes, repeated courses or prolonged treatment are necessary.

CONTINUED THERAPY

Even after completing oral therapy (such as antibiotics), ongoing topical treatment is important to prevent acne recurrence. Using multiple treatments concurrently (e.g. topical medications and oral antibiotics) is sensible because acne involves several contributing factors (e.g. excess sebum production, bacterial growth, inflammation).

SPECIFIC CIRCUMSTANCES CONCERNING ISOTRETINOIN

Isotretinoin is a powerful medication that can alter the course of acne significantly. It is used for treating severe, persistent acne that has not responded well to other treatments. It is usually taken for a defined period and may lead to long-term remission in many cases. Isotretinoin works by reducing the size of sebaceous glands and decreasing sebum production, which helps to prevent the formation of new acne lesions. It is typically prescribed for a specific duration, often ranging from several months to around six months. The treatment course is carefully monitored due to its potential side effects and the need for regular check-ups and close monitoring is necessary because of several factors (Peters 2019):

- Potential side effects: Isotretinoin can cause various side effects, some of which can be serious. These may include dryness of the skin, lips and eyes, as well as potential effects on the liver and blood lipids. Monitoring helps healthcare providers detect and manage these side effects promptly.

- Regular check-ups: Patients taking isotretinoin typically require periodic visits to their healthcare provider. During these check-ups, the provider evaluates the patient's response to treatment, monitors for any emerging side effects and adjusts the treatment plan as needed.

- Safety monitoring: Regular check-ups also ensure the safety of the treatment. They allow healthcare providers to assess how well the medication is working and to address any concerns or questions the patient may have.

IMPORTANCE OF MONITORING

Monitoring can ensure that any potential side effects are identified early and managed appropriately. Monitoring allows adjustments to the treatment plan to optimise outcomes and provides ongoing guidance and support to the patient throughout the treatment process.

LONG-TERM REMISSION

In many cases, isotretinoin can lead to long-lasting improvement or even complete clearance of acne lesions. It is known to have a prolonged effect, meaning that after completing the treatment course, some individuals may experience long-term remission from acne.

HEALTH TEACHING

Health teaching for individuals with acne vulgaris is crucial to empower them with the knowledge and strategies required to manage their condition effectively. Those who provide care and support to people with acne vulgaris are pivotal in the holistic management of care, not only addressing physical symptoms but also advising patients and dispelling common misconceptions. It is essential to communicate to patients that acne vulgaris is not caused by diet alone, including sweets or chocolate, nor is it solely due to poor hygiene; in fact, many people with acne are meticulous about their personal cleanliness.

Care providers play a critical role in ensuring patients adhere to their prescribed therapies for the full treatment course. This is vital for achieving optimal outcomes in acne vulgaris management. When isotretinoin is prescribed, particularly to those of childbearing age, it is essential to emphasise the strict requirement to avoid pregnancy due to the medication's potential to cause severe birth defects.

Empathy is a crucial component of care for patients with acne vulgaris as the emotional impact of the condition can be significant and may not always align with the severity of visible symptoms. Acne vulgaris can profoundly affect self-esteem and mental well-being and those who offer care and support should be attentive to these psychosocial aspects. Research has shown a link between severe acne and emotional distress, including suicidal ideation. While this is concerning, it highlights the importance of compassionate care and support.

Monitoring patients who are taking isotretinoin goes beyond physical assessments; it includes evaluating emotional health and mood changes. Isotretinoin can affect mood and may lead to feelings of sadness or exacerbate existing emotional challenges. In complex cases, involving general practitioners or mental health professionals in the patient's care can provide comprehensive support and ensure holistic treatment (Peters 2019).

Table 8.4 provides a list of common myths and corresponding facts about acne vulgaris.

Table 8.4 Common myths and corresponding facts about acne vulgaris

Myth	Fact
Acne is caused by poor hygiene.	Acne is primarily caused by excess oil production, clogged pores, bacteria and inflammation. While good hygiene is important, over-cleansing can aggravate acne.
Eating chocolate or greasy foods causes acne.	Diet alone does not directly cause acne. However, some individuals may find that certain foods can trigger acne flare-ups in predisposed individuals.
Popping pimples makes them go away faster.	Picking or squeezing pimples can worsen inflammation, lead to scarring and spread bacteria, prolonging the healing process.
Only teenagers get acne.	Acne can affect people of all ages, including adults. Hormonal changes, stress and certain medications can trigger acne outbreaks.
Sun exposure helps clear acne.	While sun exposure can initially dry out skin and temporarily improve acne, it can worsen acne over time by increasing oil production and causing skin damage.
Makeup causes acne.	Non-comedogenic or oil-free makeup is less likely to cause acne. Proper makeup removal and skincare routine are essential to prevent clogged pores.
Acne will go away on its own, so treatment is not necessary.	Acne can persist for years if left untreated. Early and appropriate treatment can prevent scarring and improve outcomes.
Stress does not affect acne.	Stress can trigger hormonal changes that contribute to acne flare-ups. Managing stress through relaxation techniques can help improve acne symptoms.
Acne scars will fade away naturally.	While some acne scars may improve over time, severe scars often require professional treatment such as laser therapy or chemical peels.
Acne is contagious.	Acne is not caused by bacteria that are transmitted through touch. It is a non-infectious condition influenced by internal and external factors.

Source: Adapted from Peters (2019); Stephens (2022).

Dispelling the myths with accurate information is crucial for understanding acne's causes, triggers and effective treatments. Educating oneself and others helps promote healthier skincare practices and better management of acne-related concerns. Integrating education, empathy and thorough monitoring into practice, healthcare providers can better support patients with acne vulgaris through their treatment journey, addressing both the physical and emotional aspects of the condition.

Effective health teaching for individuals with acne vulgaris involves the provision of comprehensive information and advice on skincare practices, treatment options, lifestyle modifications and psychological support.

CONCLUSION

Having an understanding of acne vulgaris is essential to care effectively for patients affected by this common dermatological condition. Acne vulgaris, characterised by various types of lesions and influenced by factors such as hormonal changes and genetic predisposition, requires a comprehensive approach to treatment and management. Mastering the principles of skincare, treatment options and the psychosocial impact of acne plays an important part in promoting effective self-care practices and supporting holistic treatment plans. Through empathy, knowledge and practical skills, those who offer care and support to people are well-positioned to make a positive impact on the lives of individuals living with acne vulgaris, ultimately contributing to improved outcomes and enhanced patient well-being.

GLOSSARY OF TERMS

Acne: A common skin condition characterised by the presence of comedones (blackheads and whiteheads), papules, pustules, nodules and cysts.

Acne vulgaris: A chronic skin condition characterised by the formation of various lesions on the skin's pilosebaceous units.

Blackhead: Also known as an open comedone, a type of acne lesion that forms when a hair follicle becomes clogged with excess sebum (oil) and dead skin cells.

Comedone: A non-inflammatory lesion caused by the clogging of a hair follicle with excess sebum and dead skin cells. Types include blackheads (open comedones) and whiteheads (closed comedones).

Cyst: A severe form of acne lesion characterised by a deep, painful, pus-filled bump under the skin.

Inflammatory lesions: Acne lesions characterised by inflammation, including papules, pustules, nodules and cysts.

Isotretinoin: A powerful oral medication used to treat severe acne that is resistant to other treatments; it reduces sebum production and prevents acne formation.

Lesion: Any abnormality in the skin's structure or function, such as comedones, papules pustules, nodules or cysts.

Nodule: A large, solid, painful acne lesion located deep within the skin.

Papule: Small, solid, raised lesion on the skin, often pink or red, caused by inflammation or infection around a hair follicle.

Pustule: Small, inflamed, pus-filled lesion on the skin, similar to a papule but with a white or yellow centre.

Sebum: The oily substance produced by sebaceous glands in the skin, which can contribute to acne when overproduced.

Sebaceous gland: Glands in the skin that produce sebum, located at the base of hair follicles.

Topical treatment: Medications applied directly to the skin to treat acne.

Whitehead: Closed comedone caused by a blocked hair follicle filled with sebum and dead skin cells under the skin's surface.

MULTIPLE CHOICE QUESTIONS

1. Which of the following is a primary characteristic of acne vulgaris?
   a) Vesicles
   b) Ulcers
   c) Comedones
   d) Wheals

2. What is the main cause of acne vulgaris?
   a) Bacterial infection
   b) Fungal infection
   c) Excessive sebum production and follicular plugging
   d) Viral infection

3. What type of comedone is characterised by an open pore with a darkened plug of sebum and dead skin cells?
   a) Whitehead
   b) Papule
   c) Nodule
   d) Blackhead

4. Where are acne vulgaris lesions most commonly found?
   a) Palms of the hands
   b) Soles of the feet
   c) Scalp
   d) Face

5. What type of lesion is a papule in acne vulgaris?
   a) Non-inflammatory
   b) Inflammatory
   c) Cystic
   d) Scar

6. What is a potential side effect of isotretinoin, an oral medication for severe acne vulgaris?
   a) Weight gain
   b) Dry skin and lips
   c) Increased appetite
   d) Hypertension

7. What hormonal changes commonly contribute to acne vulgaris in adolescents?
   a) Decreased testosterone levels
   b) Decreased oestrogen levels

c) Increased androgen levels
d) Decreased progesterone levels

8. What is the primary goal of treating acne vulgaris?
   a) Immediate scar removal
   b) Prevention of comedone formation and reduction of inflammation
   c) Permanent hair removal
   d) Reducing skin pigmentation

9. What type of lesion is a pustule in acne vulgaris?
   a) Non-inflammatory
   b) Inflammatory
   c) Cystic
   d) Scar

10. What is the term for a severe, pus-filled lesion deep within the skin in acne vulgaris?
    a) Pustule
    b) Nodule
    c) Papule
    d) Comedone

REFERENCES

American Academy of Dermatology (2024). Guidelines of care for the management of acne vulgaris. *Journal of the American Academy of Dermatology* 90 (5): 1006.e1–1006.e30. https://www.jaad.org/article/S0190-9622(23)03389-3/fulltext.

Davey, P. (2024). *Medicine at a Glance*, 5e. Oxford: Wiley.

Heng, A.H.S. and Chew, F.T. (2020). Systematic review of the epidemiology of acne vulgaris. *Scientific Reports* 10 (1): 5754. doi: 10.1038/s41598-020-62715-3.

Leung, A.K., Barankin, B., Lam, J.M. et al. (2021). Dermatology: how to manage acne vulgaris. *Drugs Context* 10: 2021-8-6. doi: 10.7573/dic.2021-8-6.

Peate, I. (2019). *Fundamentals of Assessment and Care Planning for Nurses*. Oxford: Wiley.

Peters, J. (2019). Nursing patients with skin disorders (Chapter 13). In: *Alexander's Nursing Practice*, 5e (ed. I. Peate). London: Elsevier.

Primary Care Dermatology Society (2023). Acne vulgaris. https://www.pcds.org.uk/patient-info-leaflets/acne-vulgaris (accessed June 2024).

Stephens, M. (2022). The person with a skin disorder (Chapter 35). In: *Nursing Practice*, 3e (ed. I. Peate and A. Mitchell). Oxford: Wiley.

Waldman, A., Bolotin, D., Arndt, K.A. et al. (2017). ASDS guidelines task force: consensus recommendations regarding the safety of lasers, dermabrasion, chemical peels, energy devices, and skin surgery during and after isotretinoin use. *Dermatologic Surgery* 43 (10): 1249–1262.

Weller, R.B., Hunter, H.A., and Mann, M.W. (2014). *Clinical Dermatology*, 5e. Oxford: Wiley.

MCQ Answers

Chapter 1   Anatomy and Physiology of the Skin

1. (b); 2. (c); 3. (b); 4. (c); 5. (a); 6. (c); 7. (b); 8. (d); 9. (d); 10. (b).

Chapter 2   Assessment of the Skin

1. (b); 2. (b); 3. (c); 4. (a); 5. (c); 6. (a); 7. (a); 8. (b); 9. (b); 10. (a).

Chapter 3   Psoriasis

1. (b); 2. (b); 3. (c); 4. (b); 5. (c); 6. (d); 7. (d); 8. (c); 9. (b); 10. (c).

Chapter 4   Eczema

1. (c); 2. (d); 3. (c); 4. (c); 5. (c); 6. (c); 7. (b); 8. (c); 9. (c); 10. (b).

Chapter 5   Melanoma

1. (c); 2. (c); 3. (c); 4. (b); 5. (b); 6. (b); 7. (c); 8. (a); 9. (d); 10. (c).

Chapter 6   Burns

1. (b); 2. (c); 3. (c); 4. (b); 5. (b); 6. (b); 7. (a); 8. (b); 9. (c); 10. (b).

Chapter 7   Herpes Zoster

1. (b); 2. (c); 3. (c); 4. (b); 5. (a); 6. (b); 7. (b); 8. (b); 9. (b); 10. (d).

Chapter 8   Acne Vulgaris

1. (c); 2. (c); 3. (d); 4. (d); 5. (b); 6. (b); 7. (c); 8. (b); 9. (b); 10. (b).

Index

Note: Page numbers in *italics* and **bold** refer to figures and tables, respectively.